"You don't have to have eati addiction to benefit from this s remarkable and holistic appro… much has been left out to assist the reader to come to a better understanding of self and life process, communication of Divine through our bodies and our connection to Super Consciousness, highlighting the role of the "free will" that each one of us possesses, the importance of self reverence and self value."

"The third millennium is indeed about shifting to higher awareness, a time to resolve belief systems and perceptions that no longer serve us. The simple applications of Monica's book will no doubt take the reader into a new reality or paradigm which will be paramount in successfully processing the present shift into a more promising and peaceful future... and it all starts with self."

Rose Saroyan - Bio-Energy Therapist

"A very thought-inspiring personal journey but one to which anyone of all ages can relate whether partially or entirely. The search for one's own healthy calm and essence is very much worth the time spent reading this candid conversation between the reader and the author. "

Hennie Cheah – Educator

"It is rare to find a book that risks such intimacy in the sharing of a personal journey; I felt inspired and nurtured along the way. The clear presentation of the wisdom gained, offered as a series of "Ways", along with doable applications, compelled me to experiment with them in my own life. A delightful, practical and helpful book."

**Cathy McPherson -
Manager of Mental Health Services,
Hamilton Family Health Team, Ontario**

Get Your Inner Power Back!

BLUEPRINT TO STOP BINGE EATING TAKING OVER
YOUR LIFE WHILE RECONNECTING WITH YOUR SOUL

Monica Villarreal

BALBOA.
PRESS

A DIVISION OF HAY HOUSE

Balboa Press books may be ordered through booksellers or by contacting:

Balboa Press
A Division of Hay House
1663 Liberty Drive
Bloomington, IN 47403
www.balboapress.com
1-(877) 407-4847

Because of the dynamic nature of the Internet, any web addresses or
links contained in this book may have changed since publication and
may no longer be valid. The views expressed in this work are solely those
of the author and do not necessarily reflect the views of the publisher,
and the publisher hereby disclaims any responsibility for them.

The author of this book does not dispense medical advice or prescribe the use
of any technique as a form of treatment for physical, emotional, or medical
problems without the advice of a physician, either directly or indirectly. The
intent of the author is only to offer information of a general nature to help
you in your quest for emotional and spiritual well-being. In the event you use
any of the information in this book for yourself, which is your constitutional
right, the author and the publisher assume no responsibility for your actions.

Any people depicted in stock imagery provided by Thinkstock are models,
and such images are being used for illustrative purposes only.
Certain stock imagery © Thinkstock.

ISBN: 978-1-4525-3279-0 (sc)
ISBN: 978-1-4525-3280-6 (e)

Printed in the United States of America
Balboa Press rev. date: 4/26/2011

To Ricardo, my loving companion
in the adventure of life.

Contents

Preface

1978. It is about 9:00pm and the kitchen is dark. We had supper about an hour ago and mom and dad are upstairs reading and watching a TV program. The house is quiet but inside me it is not. I am thinking over and over again about "that" delicious bread my dad brought from our favorite bakery ... a local bakery located near the hospital where he works and which every single day sees freshly baked loafs of bread flying out the door. Sometimes they barely make it from the oven to the shelves!

Gathering my thoughts and visions I go to the kitchen and open the pantry door, turn on the light and climb onto the shelf to be able to reach the bag which is... Up there! While I am climbing, I remember that there is also this super tasty orange marmalade that has little delicate rinds in it and think about how really well it would go with the bread and homemade butter that is in the fridge. Hmmm, my mouth is watering by now and I cannot wait to put them all together. I am 9 years old, have a slim frame, tons of freckles and more than plenty of curly and unruly hair that my mom finds so hard to control that it often drives her crazy. She hates seeing me with all this hair in my face and not being able to see my eyes.

As soon as I reach the bag, I undo it, leaving it wide open, get the marmalade, the butter and a knife and position myself in front of it all to start my feast, right there in the pantry. I cannot wait to taste these glorious foods. I start diving into the bag and eat three or four buns with generous amounts of butter and marmalade. It feels good to me. I feel like I'm in heaven. I think that my whole being is happy now.

This became a routine for me and I wonder if my mom ever noticed the "disappearing" buns. It is a shame that I cannot ask her because she has already passed away. I wonder if she suspected it was me or if she thought it was my brother, my dad or perhaps the live-in maid. I do not recall hearing anything about it.

As I grew up I became very fond of all kinds of cakes, chocolate brownies, chocolate glaze, crackers filled with cream, ice cream and so on. By my early twenties I had fallen in love with something I discovered on my frequent trips to Miami after I became a flight attendant: key lime pie. Every time I landed in Miami I "had" to have a slice of key lime pie. In no time and with little effort I gained about 20 pounds and looked quite full and rounded. I continued devouring sweets here and there and since for the most part I ate healthily, didn't drink or smoke, I thought I was doing just fine but, by my mid-twenties, I started to feel very tired, nauseated, dizzy and even fainted several times. No, I was not pregnant, although my father had thought of that. A 4 hour blood glucose test revealed that I had a serious case of hypoglycemia. I stopped eating sweets cold turkey because I was scared that I would become diabetic and perhaps experience a diabetic coma. I lost 10 pounds in the first week and some more afterwards. For five years I didn't touch sugar and also limited my intake of carbs. After that I reintroduced them slowly into my diet and ate them a bit sporadically with no evident side effects.

I went on like this for some years but in 2007, while eating out, I started to have a bit more, and a bit more each time. What I thought I had under control was getting out of control again. I was not aware of it because it was gradual and I was not fainting or feeling sick. Time passed by and summer arrived. By then I started experiencing hormonal imbalances, which I had never had before, and then little by little, all sorts of symptoms showed up: digestive problems, food allergies and intolerance, weight loss, extreme fatigue, generalized body pain, insomnia, irritability, anxiety, panic attacks, eye pain, and loss of motivation, concentration and focus. By the end of 2008 I had lost 22 pounds–and that was not the end of it. By that time my stomach was barely accepting water. I would get bloated and experience heartburn easily so herbal teas were my best friends for a while. What I was eating was mostly vegetarian and I became very fond of light soups and congees, even for breakfast. I was also eating gluten-free and raw foods and doing some juicing. (You will be able to read more in detail my whole three year journey in the latter part of the book.)

It Came Back!

It is March, 2009. It is Saturday, 8:30 pm. My husband is upstairs chilling out watching a movie, and I am in the kitchen finishing the dishes. After I am done, I remember that I have these amazingly soft and fresh dates in the refrigerator and I reach for the box. There are about twelve of them and while standing up with the box open in front of me I eat them all in a frenzy. I was not planning to have them all but as I finished the first one I wanted another one, and another one and so on. It felt as if I had this hole inside me with no bottom. I did not get any signs of fullness but I was aware enough to realize that something odd was happening. Anyhow, the dates were delicious–and gone in a flash. I turned off the light, went upstairs and put the whole thing into the back of my mind for the rest of the evening. "Mañana (tomorrow)", I thought, "I will go back to thinking about it."

I did not bother with it the next day but after a few days I went through another binge episode. This time the prey was a whole bag of Brazil nuts. There were 2 handfuls in the bag which is a lot for Brazil nuts. I grabbed the bag but this time I took the time to sit down, and started digging into it. Each Brazil nut took me to the heavens once more. Despite the fact that I had eaten more than a dozen, I found it curious that I didn't feel heavy or sick with all that fat. I thought, "Hmmm, it seems that I still have this deep, hard-to-fill hole inside me!"

At this point I knew that that something beyond or combined with a physical cause was happening again. For the last few years I had been reading and learning a great deal about personal evolution and spiritual growth and at the same time letting go of many old hurts and energies, so I thought, "There must be something deeper here wanting to be healed." I decided to step back and become the observer of myself; see myself eating and delving into the deep emotions I was experiencing without labeling the situation or myself; simply allow myself to be in that very moment and to experience the situation with all my senses.

Strong cravings for sweets and nuts continued for a week or two and although I mostly resisted, many times I ate a bit of them. I kept doing the exercise of being very present at the moment. I would eat slowly and savor every bite of whatever it was but it did not take me too long to suspect that I was going through a serious case of Candida overgrowth.

Candida feeds off sugar, flour and carbs in general and that was precisely what I was craving more and more. I did some research on my own and found that I had pretty much all the symptoms associated with it so in April 2009 I decided to embark on a new healing journey that would take me through different Candida cleanses until I got to a diet that made sense to me. Since summer 2007 when I felt that my body was changing (see "Health Mystery" for my full story), I had been seeing all sorts of natural health care practitioners including energy healers, nutritionists, chi gung masters, reflexologists, angel therapists, etc. Each step of the way had already been intense but every single person I consulted helped me in one way or another to put the pieces together although none of them told me, before I suspected it, that I was experiencing Candida overgrowth. I guess I had to get to that conclusion on my own while reaching the edge of a cliff, a point where I felt deep down, "This is it. I have to make a decision to live, right here and now, or this will not turn out well!"

This took place in winter 2009 when I had reached 88 pounds, looked quite emaciated and felt very empty inside. I was wearing size 12 Junior and three layers of clothes to stay warm.

In any event, looking back I appreciate that every single person helped me in a different way when I most needed it and when I did not have the strength to do it by myself. All was perfect and appropriate and contributed immensely to my personal and spiritual evolution. Today, it seems like a far-away dream but it is wonderful to realize how strong, resilient, wise and capable the body and spirit can be.

In short, what I started to experience back in 2007 was much more than physical imbalances or Candida overgrowth. It was a real and clear opportunity that my whole being was giving me to expand and evolve; to move to higher levels of awareness. This developed into a deep experience to heal my body, mind and spirit. I think that it had to hit me at my weakest point—food and specially sweets. It had to come with a façade, the façade of what is known as Candida. That was the manifestation, that's all.

The whole process I went through was always filled with multiple trials and errors and small and big triumphs and disappointments. It served me to dig out lots of old stuff that was cluttering me inside and causing a spiritual constipation. It allowed me to realize how, old, and non-serving beliefs were affecting my experience of life. Thanks to this journey my perspective of life (and me in it of course) expanded. I came to realize that I have the power to choose every single moment from a place of inner power and unconditional love. I discovered that true healing happens from the inside out and that it all starts with making the decision to choose life.

I also realized that it does not have to be a dreadful or a scary process, but that it can be very practical and occasionally even fun. I found out that there is no need to pay thousands of dollars in healing therapies; neither to spend thousands of hours to see small measurable results. All you need is you and you have it all inside. With the aid of simple practices or exercises you can take yourself to the next level, then to the next and so on. Again, the most important thing is to make the choice and whatever you do, do it with love and full awareness.

I think it is exciting to realize that each of us has access to a wealth of wisdom and resources that can help us to achieve new understandings, to clear blocking energies, to heal old hurts and wounds, and to feel worthy, vibrant, joyful and connected with our soul again.

After all I went through these past three years, all I experimented with, and the different results I obtained, I think it is time to share with you and others my own story and the practical lessons I have learned from the journey.

It is my wish to be open and honest with you and let you know that no matter how dark the place seems to be where you are right now, you can get out of it with grace and courage. I did it. You can do it too.

It is also my wish that the recollection of simple, useful and enjoyable ways to overcome binge eating and food obsessions presented here serve you well beyond your imagination. I have tested them all and have lived their benefits within my own skin. Still do. I encourage you to be open, to try each of them and adapt them to your own style and preferences as you go along. Experiment with them, have fun, be creative! Follow your intuition and trust that you can do this if you really, really want to. Also remember to be patient, that everything has its own time and rhythm and that this experience you are having will pass too.

One last thing before we dive into the ways–you do not have to implement them all at once. Pick one and practise it for a few weeks. Then pick another one and do the same. With time your own inner guidance will tell you what to do in a given moment, just like that.

Awareness

To be aware means to be conscious and the most important awareness there is to be practised is awareness of the self. Self-awareness is one of the pillars of personal evolution, self-realization and complete freedom. It allows you to recognize who you are and become conscious of your emotions, thoughts, beliefs, preferences, motivations, actions and behavior patterns.

Self-awareness is one of the keys to opening up the gates that allow entry into your soul, and release what is blocking you, what is holding you back and keeping you in a non-enjoyable, detrimental cycle. The cycle of eating beyond what your body needs (especially sweets and flour), then feeling guilty, ashamed and even sick, and afterwards indulging in food again because you are not feeling happy with yourself. Self-awareness helps to cut the cord of "What the heck, I'll have another piece." It shatters the belief that you need to eat that cake and get instant satisfaction otherwise you are going to perish.

Yes, in order to break this never ending, exhausting cycle, self-awareness needs to be in place. But how can you practise it on the spur of the moment when you are a few seconds away from gobbling down that amazing chocolate cake with creamy chocolate glaze and all?

Application:

First of all STOP. Make the conscious decision to stop before you start diving into the cake and take a deep, belly breath. I know. You feel that you cannot wait to slice the cake with the fork and put a piece into your mouth, but you know what? You can wait a few seconds if you decide to. Just try it. Stop, breathe deeply and observe the cake, smell it, feel it, and also see and feel yourself right there, in front of it about to eat it. You have to become an observer at a distance watching yourself. Notice your hand holding the fork; notice your emotions, your thoughts, your body, the anxiety for eating the whole thing without anybody stopping you. Notice all the details you can about <u>this</u> specific moment and then, if you feel that you have to have it, start eating it without losing the focus on the cake and YOU eating the cake, savoring it. To increase your awareness even further stay...

Fully Present

When you are fully present you are fully living. You are noticing the details of what is going on and savoring life with all your senses. You more easily open up to let in insights and ideas that can bring you clarity and new understanding.

How many times, while you are eating, have you noticed that your mind jumps from one thought to another, and to the next, and then to another one? Your mind incessantly reminds you of the laundry you have not picked up, the call you forgot to make, the letter you have to mail, the dress you have to buy, etc.

From now on, and this is something that gets better with practice, make the decision to stay present, even if thoughts pass by, notice them too; without judging them or worrying about what you are thinking. When the time to eat comes, no matter what it is, become an observer and stay present in the moment with the food, the environment, and yourself. Feel the cutlery in your hand, notice the colors and shapes of the food, smell its aroma, feel its texture in your mouth, sense the flavors with your taste buds, and notice how you feel, how your body feels and where it feels what.

Also notice what you want to eat first, and what emotions are going through you. It is about being there and simply allowing oneself to be immersed in the wonderful act of eating. You will be amazed at how, spontaneously, with no extra effort, you start becoming more and more aware of yourself, your emotions and your patterns. This simple practice will open the door to you and take you to a new land of revelations and aha! moments that in time will set you free from food obsessions and binge eating.

It happens gradually and with its own rhythm. The beauty of this is that you do not have to force anything, to push away anything, to pull anything! No more struggle with yourself. It all unfolds naturally in front of your eyes if you allow it, and you start recognizing that your relationship with food, the way you feel about it starts to change and that you start to experience more motivation to do other interesting things, things that you love beside eating and binging!

Application:

About three years ago I made the conscious decision to practice "being fully present", as much as possible. I say as much as possible because in the beginning it is easy to forget and just go about mindlessly with whatever you are doing. To me it is challenging for example to be fully present when I have limited time to accomplish something and I am rushing into it. Anyway, I decided to try it and to help myself in the beginning by doing a simple exercise. It consisted of telling myself what I was doing each single moment. This helped me to focus on the now and be fully present with my actions and emotions.

For example, if I was dressing in the morning I would say to myself, "I'm putting my pants on" and while I was actually doing it I would watch myself doing it and feel my legs one by one sliding into the pants. If I was washing dishes I would say to myself, "I'm rinsing the dishes with warm water" and would pay close attention to all that was happening. I would feel the warm water running through my fingers, notice the bubbles, hear the water flowing, and so on. If I was gobbling down some Brazil nuts, I would tell myself, "I am eating these Brazil nuts" and would chew each of them slowly, feeling them in my mouth, getting their flavor and smelling their aroma, while watching myself at a distance, with no judgment, just observing my act of eating with no restraint.

I have to confess that in general I found this a tough practice because I am a person who likes to be on the go most of the time; to get things done in the least time possible. I tend to like dressing, speaking, walking, eating, and working fast! Being fully present meant to slow down, relax, and allow myself to be a participant in each moment with all my senses.

This practice not only helped me to be more present each instant but also allowed me to realize that I had an unhealthy sense of urgency, one that had false beliefs attached to it. For example, I recognized that I had a strong feeling of not having enough time to do all the things I wanted to do, and that this feeling was quite overwhelming. Eating fast as if time was going to take away my food, rushing through the house chores as if I was missing the fun I could have when not doing them, working 14-16 hours a day to accomplish all my dreams in less time, were normal things for me. One day I realized that it was not only about time–it was about a belief I had that, "there was not enough". And I was applying it to time, food, health and other things. In the case of food I was feeling that I had to eat it all at once, as much as I could because, "what if tomorrow I do not have it." This belief fed my need for binge eating and served as an excuse too.

Slowing down helped me to appreciate life as it is and value its own natural course. It also helped me to understand that I have plenty of time, and food, and opportunities to do all of what I want to do. I am now moving at a much slower pace but I have to tell you that still at times the "rushing mode" tries to creep back in and get me into its game. But now, I quickly notice and say to myself, "Breathe ... Slow down ... I have plenty of everything ... All is well". And this helps like magic .

Feelings and Emotions

As a human being you are have something beautiful that allows you to experience life in a unique way, and which serves you as a compass too – emotion.

Most of us are afraid of feeling certain things such as pain, sadness, depression, anger, guilt, frustration, and jealousy because they feel unpleasant, or we have been taught they are "bad".

The truth is that an emotion is simply a form of energy being expressed which can serve different purposes: it can make you feel alive, alert you, guide you, help you make more conscious choices, evolve, etc.

Now, food and emotions... hmmm ... They are very well interconnected! Have you noticed that we humans put lots of emphasis on food? We love to go to events where there is food. We eat to celebrate. We eat if we feel sad, frustrated, bored, anxious, depressed, guilty, etc.

Many of us, since we were little got this message that food is associated with pleasure, reward and/or punishment. I remember my parents telling me things like: "Clear you plate or you cannot leave the table... there are millions of children dying every day of hunger." Also, they would say things like: "Good girl! Let's go for an ice cream". I also remember that in my house there was some kind of mystery around food. My mom used to buy "fancy" snacks and imported foods for "those special occasions", which meant friends and family visiting us and lock them in a separate pantry. I knew where the key was because she told me but I also knew that this food was "very special" and not meant to be devoured by me or anyone else without my mom's OK. I remember that at times I would feel like eating something different, something "fun", from that pantry and I would say: "Mom, I want to eat something delicious" and most of the time the answer I would get would be something like: "Make yourself a cheese sandwich or a fruit punch." It would be very rare that the vault containing those exotic goodies would open for me or for us unless it was a special occasion. This may seem like a little normal thing but it was sending a clear message that we were not special enough to have these things.

Let me say that my mom and dad were strong in character and quite disciplinary people but also they were very loving, giving and dedicated parents. I know in my heart they did their best. As they say: "they didn't know better". They had their own beliefs, limitations and challenges—as all of us do—and subconsciously were passing them to us, their children.

As I grew up I became very interested in nutrition and natural health and with time became more and more conscious of my eating habits, but sweets were also my soft spot. It is funny how I always thought that I did not have any vice; I did not smoke, drink, do drugs or anything like that. It never occurred to me that indulging in sweets with no control was an out of balance behavior, until the day I fainted and I realized the consequences. As I mentioned before, by my mid-twenties I had abused my body with so many sorts of sweet treats and pastries that my body spoke loud and clear. It started giving me clues such as fainting. After I broke the habit overnight, I embarked on a fifteen-year search for the most reliable information available on healthy eating and lifestyle. I experimented with all kinds of diets and body-mind disciplines and became someone known for my knowledge in this area. Friends would come to me to ask me about food ... what to eat and not to eat to be healthy, to lose weight, to gain energy to sleep well, etc. Little did I know that while I was thinking that I had the answers, I was getting trapped in my own game; my own laboratory where I thought I had everything under control.

Well, at least that is what I thought. But the day came when I had to face another story. After having mastered the principles of health, vitality and longevity, and applied them all with visible success for almost fifteen years, one day, in the year of 2007, I found myself experiencing loss of energy and motivation, hormonal imbalances, sleep problems, indigestion, constipation and generalized pain among other things. My health was going downhill rapidly for no apparent reason and I found myself being forced to going on another quest for the truth.

My experiences in the past three years have helped me to see that the main issue was not really in my biology (although I had to go through a chronic candida overgrowth that took me to a point where I was losing it fast). These obvious things were just a façade behind which deeper issues were lurking, waiting to be taken to the light and resolved. I came to understand that I had been holding a thick layer of pent-up emotions waiting to erupt like a furious volcano and be dealt with once and for all. I finally realized not without surprise the depth and kind of dark emotions I had buried inside me: anger, guilt, grief and unworthiness were the main ones.

I am spending a bit more time on this chapter because expressing emotions is one of the things that some human beings find difficult, and without expressing our emotions we cannot achieve balance or lead a healthy life. It is hard for many to express, especially, those considered negative emotions. In general we are taught to not express anger, hatred, resentment and frustration. Or … do you remember a time when your parents said to you: "It's OK to feel furious. It is safe. Let yourself experience it." If you do, excellent! I do not.

So for me, food, and more than anything, sweets, became an escape and a way to numb myself, to quiet my emotions and my spirit, to fit in and feel accepted. Eating sweets and binging also gave me a sense of power, of being in control, because food cannot argue with you, can it? Food just follows your command. It does not criticize you or tell you what to do next. It is easy to feel in control with food and that is one of the reasons it is difficult to let it go too. Because it means letting go of control, the need to be on command and basically face and trust the person you are and what you feel.

This recent health experience helped me to see that I had all these "undigested" emotions and a big desire to feel that I was finally in control. In the process my digestive system took the punch and without me being conscious of it, I started to **somatize**; to put psychological and emotional distress into physical symptoms right there in my digestive system. What I had not been able to digest mentally now I was not able to digest physically. Interesting, eh?

This was an opportunity for me to go through the undigested lot of emotions that had been waiting to be released so that I could start nourishing my whole being with new understandings and truths, and move into higher levels of consciousness. In a nutshell, I was presented with the opportunity to learn and evolve.

For over two years I cried my eyes out until they almost melted. I recalled memories that would make me burst into tears in a snap; no matter where I was, or what I was doing (eating, walking, taking a shower, talking, sleeping) I would cry with ease. I noticed that the more I allowed it to happen, spontaneously, the better I felt. Also, I could sense that my physical health was taking a turn for the better as time passed. This process helped me to gain clarity and understand why at times I would feel unworthy and left out, feel this uncomfortable rush going on inside to do, to be, to gather, to eat it all while I could, so I did not miss out!

I understood why I felt anger when seeing others eating certain foods that were not agreeing with me that very moment. I now comprehend why I felt like a rebel without a cause ... Having a strong willed spirit I had negative feelings towards the fact that my parents restricted me and controlled me too much. Having a special pantry locked at home and every year getting very cheap (nothing special) school utensils had given me the impression that I was not good enough to get and enjoy the fine things in life.

Having to dread the fact, when I was in elementary school, that my lunch box was always full of smelly, home-made foods such as guava juice and rice with ground meat, made me believe that I was different, that I could not fit in; that I was not deserving of fun foods that came in colorful packages. Today I appreciate big time that my mom wanted me to be healthy but in those days I felt ashamed, out of place. I don't think she ever imagined how I felt and we never spoke about it. I was never open with her anyway; somehow I felt apprehensive about expressing these things. I was a Marco Polo type of girl, wanting to explore, discover, and have adventures all the time and would clash with the precise order and discipline my mom and dad wanted to instill in me. I know that discipline is something very important to learn in the early years but I think they were so worried about my free and innocent spirit that they did not know another way to contain me.

Food, as I said before, became the perfect escape, and sweets the most preferred way to get the sweetness of life from the outside world. I had these feelings of deprivation inside me that needed compensation for all I had not enjoyed until this point so... let's bring on the banquet!

But after years of overindulging in sweets and pastries during my childhood and early youth I started to experience hypoglycemia and I became conscious that I had to correct this course otherwise I could become diabetic, a condition I feared a great deal. I opted for cutting out all sweets cold turkey and reduce dramatically my intake of flour and starches. I had built in the "chip of discipline" so doing it that way was not a problem. I became a super healthy and conscious eater, and very savvy about nutrition. Some people would say a purist. This went well for years until one day, three years ago, a new health crisis hit me, manifesting itself through a weak point of mine... my love for sweets! To me it was as if my spirit was saying, "OK, this is enough; there are still issues to be resolved and hard discipline is not really the way to deal with them. The problem is not the sweets; the real issues are still inside you and it is time for resolution".

Application:

Since I learned firsthand how important it is to feel and express my emotions fully, and understood that no matter how dark or painful they are (whether a physical pain or a heated emotion), they cannot annihilate me or break me apart, I have been doing the conscious exercise of allowing myself to feel whatever comes to me, right there, with my whole being, and if involves another person, express it to him or her calmly.

Whenever I find myself feeling something that catches my attention, either an uncomfortable physical sensation or a strong emotion, I embrace it instead of repressing it. I stay with it and do my best to not label it, judge it, manipulate it or push it away. I simply let it be and at the same time take a few deep, belly breaths to allow it to go through me. With this I give it permission to be, to express in my body and also resolve. At times it feels exacerbating, more painful and profound but this is what helps such an emotion or sensation to continue its path and not get trapped in your being! It is amazing to experience this. It is incredible to feel the intensity and then feel how it unfolds and evaporates by itself. It works, believe me, it does. And although a particular dark emotion or pain may come back more than once, each time it does and you allow it to be it appears with less power so you feel it less overwhelmingly.

I have applied this principle to eating as well. For more than a year I have felt lots of anxiety associated with eating. I felt anxious and even hyperventilated right before starting to eat, whether it was a regular healthy meal or something not that "ideal" for me that moment like... chocolate! I would get this feeling that I could not wait for too long, that I was approaching the end of my rope and I had to put that food into my mouth. I could also see that if I had to wait for whatever reason I would feel irritable and even mad. There was a strong charge of dense energy in me, anxiety and I even felt a sensation behind my right thigh, in the muscle, as if something was grabbing me there and not letting go; like a bite. I became aware of this regular occurrence and instead of pushing it away (as much as I wanted), I decided to embrace it and feel it in my core, breathing deeply and slowly, giving it the chance to resolve in its own time, and allowing it to continue its way . By doing this I provided a safe space to clear these things out until one day they did not come back any more.

The other example I would like to share with you is related to cravings and the feelings of fear, sadness, anger, boredom or anxiety. My cravings for sugary foods and pastries would intensify a great deal when something made me feel any of these emotions; when I had an argument with someone close to me, or someone pushed my buttons I immediately felt like retreating and having something sweet, comforting. At the beginning I gave into it many times, but always tried to be very present with what I was doing and feeling. So as time passed, and I kept practising the simple principles outlined in this book, I was able to stop in my tracks, take distance and see the game I was about to play once again.

I was able to stay with the uncomfortable emotion and accept it totally reassuring myself that it was OK, that it was safe to feel it. That this emotion was part of me too and that it was not going to kill me or make me weaker. I also reminded myself of what was really, really important to me, and that I was much more than this emotion. That love started with myself and that this was an opportunity to demonstrate it.

With time, practice and patience, I became more conscious of the fact that ultimately it was my decision, my choice, no matter how ugly the world was looking out there, or how much I wanted to place the responsibility on others. I was able to gauge the consequences of what I was about to do, for my body and my soul, and tell myself things like: "Been there, done that; I know how it is and it is not that great so… why bother!!"

At some point in the past I thought I was a "victim" of food obsessions and food addictions but finally the time came when my light bulb came on! I realized that as a human being with divine essence that never dies, I had the power to choose whatever I wanted, and that the rest was based on false belief systems and misconceptions I had acquired in the past.

Being present, and allowing myself to feel and experience my emotions without holding back (while taking some deep, deep breaths), opened the doors for me to new understandings and a renewed concept of myself... I stopped looking at me as small and powerless!

Now, let's talk about what I have been repeatedly mentioning and which can be one of your best allies in this process and in life ...

Breathing

Breathing is free, available to all and it is very, very powerful – more than you think, I bet.

How many of us take at least a couple of conscious breaths a day?

Conscious breathing is underrated. Although breathing techniques are taught by many people who teach yoga, Chi Gung and meditation, it seems to me that the magnitude of conscious breathing is not really understood. Conscious breathing is one of the things that helped me to become a more balanced and healthier person in many ways. Conscious breathing is in itself a tool that we all have access to, at any time, and which can help you to accomplish things that some would consider miraculous, like healing the body. When you consciously breathe you take in air slowly, you feel how your lungs, stomach and even your cells expand and receive air, and life!

One single conscious breath can help your body to unlock trapped energies, release toxins of a physical or an emotional nature, rejuvenate and balance itself. Breathing means life and acceptance.

Application:

By now you know very well that I am all into deep breathing and have given you some examples on when to use it. I couple of years ago I finally grasped the level importance of deep and conscious breathing when a Chi Gung master taught me a simple breathing practice that I did for almost a year, four times a day (upon awakening, before lunch, before dinner and before going to sleep), and for 5 minutes or so. Conscious breathing helped me immensely to improve my digestion, calm down in the middle of a panic attack, move stocked energy within me, boost my energy levels, and regain control of my health. The breathing I used to do was like this: I would take a deep breath, slowly, counting up to seven, feeling my stomach going up; then I would hold it for four seconds and then I would exhale, slowly, counting up to ten while feeling my stomach flattening.

After that year, and as I got healthier, I started to cut down the many routines I had adopted and this included this specific way of breathing. I was feeling stronger and my inner wisdom was telling me to opt for simplicity so I decided to go back to the basics.

Today, deep breathing is something I still practise but with no agenda. I make sure I take some conscious breaths here and there, expand and receive life and balance with each breath and that's it. Breathing is what keeps us alive, right? Well, deep, conscious breathing helps you to go beyond a mere existence. It opens you up unblocking obstructing energies; it releases your own body's powers to balance your physiology, emotions and soul. Each deep conscious breath helps to confirm you are opting for life! So breathe amigo … breathe away, feel how your body takes in the air and allows life to fill you up from top to bottom and front to back.

One simple deep breath is a meditation in itself. It has the power to ground you and put you at ease. Try it!

Forgive Yourself & Others

I cannot emphasize enough the act of forgiveness. Forgiveness, starting with forgiving yourself is vital to cut the cords that chain you to undesirable habits. I implore you to take this practice to heart and do it diligently. I know… we all have a long list of "should haves" and "could haves". And yes, perhaps you could have done it better and maybe you shouldn't have done "that". It doesn't matter anymore. Past is past and it was an experience, treat it as such. How much energy do you think it is taking away from you in the present? Don't you think that this energy would be better spent in loving yourself, accepting yourself and allowing yourself to experiment with new fresh ideas and new ways of being – now that you know better? Take what you learned from it, forgive yourself and move on. You will see how much lighter you feel.

Did somebody do something to you that you think was unfair and hurtful? Are you holding onto old grudges or wounds? Most likely they didn't have a clue how to do it differently. And if they did do something on purpose be sure that they did it from a place of hurt and fear. In any case, it is time to let go of that and stop defining yourself for what they did or they did not do to you, or for what you could have done or avoided doing. It is time to stop feeling responsible for other people's acts, or feeling like a victim. Life happens. The ups and downs are part of life and who has not had their own share?

Now you are in a different place living your own life and wanting to blossom beautifully. You are you, only you and not they. You are you and not their actions or false beliefs. They did what they could with what they had to offer. If you can see this with an open heart, forgive them (and forgive yourself), and then choose focusing on the present moment. Trust me that you will have more clarity of mind, energy and freedom to enjoy your life on your own terms and food will not be the "drug" you need to numb yourself or to punish yourself anymore.

Application:

At the beginning of 2009 when I was uncovering some old wounds related to my childhood I realized that I was holding deep down a cocktail of emotions including guilt for not having grieved my mom fully when she passed away (I was 17 years old and in my peak of rebellion). I was full of resentment for not having had the opportunity to enjoy her company longer–and have the chance to go over the bumpy early and teenage years and develop a tranquil, meaningful adult relationship. So, I decided to write letters and burn them.

I wrote letters to my mom where I expressed my feelings about those days of continuous fighting over little, silly things, that in any case hurt me, and also wrote some to my father and grandma who have passed away too. I even wrote letters to my siblings with the intention of clearing any lingering unresolved issue and lastly, I wrote to myself.

At times I would go to the lake and sit on the stones and burn the letters there. I even wrote a few while there. While they were burning I made the choice of letting go what was not honoring me any more whether I knew what it was or not… you do not have to know it all; it is enough as long as you open your heart and give yourself permission to release those heavy energies. By the way, these are letters that you do not have to share with anyone if you do not want to. And the beauty of it is that it works because it is all about you, nobody else!

You may repeat this healing exercise as many times as you feel. And if you find writing too much work, sit down and talk to each person you want to forgive. Imagine she or he is there and simply say whatever comes to mind. Be prepared with a box of tissues, and let it all hang out!

A day will come when you look at these memories with other lenses, even with a smile on your face. The resentment, anger, jealousy, guilt, whatever it is, gets replaced with love, understanding and compassion. You will see… you will see. The act of forgiveness will help you to regain the balance you are craving for, and the way you see and choose food won't be the same anymore.

Self-Talk

Talking to oneself is free, fun and extremely powerful. It is one of those things that you have to experience to realize how valuable and effective it can be. And I am not referring to affirmations or any kind of repetitions. They are quite mechanical and lack of one key ingredient that is emotion … the heart. Most people get tired of doing affirmations after a while and give up because it becomes a chore and many times the results are far from what they desire. I can tell you that there is a huge difference between repeating like a parrot the same sentence over and over again and talking to yourself, from the heart, with full emotion. I have tried both and even though I obtained results (limited) with affirmations, I am no longer using them because I have discovered the real power of talking to myself in a more personal and intimate way.

I say, you can skip affirmations for a while (if you do those) and try talking to yourself, as if you were talking to a friend that you love dearly. The idea is to create a bond, a healthy and honest relationship with yourself, the same way you do with other people. You can use self-talk to reassure or praise yourself–to express yourself gratitude. To

The

Monica Villarreal

talk about how you are feeling in a given moment or to ask yourself about something you want to know. Also, you might ask yourself if there is anything you need to know about a specific thing or in general. There are no rules or limitations to this.

When it comes to food and you are eating beyond what your body really needs, for example, it is a great idea to talk with yourself and ask some questions such as: "Why am I doing this?" "What are you (habit) trying to tell me?" "Why are you coming back again, and again?" "Is this who I truly am?"

Ask whatever comes to your mind that may lead to more clarity and keep quiet, breathing deeply. Trust yourself and be ready to get the answer at any moment… No need for brain power or arm twisting. Your inner wisdom will deliver it to you in its own way … it could be in a dream!

The more you do this the better you get at it, and the more natural and comfortable you feel with it. This exercise will allow you to get important insights on what is going on behind the façade of binge eating – or any other pattern. It is a simple and friendly practice that does not need much, just you. It will help you to understand yourself better to make more conscious choices which in turn will free you up from upsetting behavior patterns that you are willing to let go.

Application:

I have grown quite fond of talking to myself and I have discovered that it can be very refreshing and fun. I do it very often in a natural and spontaneous way as I go about the day.

In the beginning you may feel silly and you will tend to forget but as you become your own observer, and best friend, and start communicating with yourself more and more you will feel more comfortable with it and you will be happily

26

surprised of how valuable talking to yourself is. Talking to yourself is the fast way to establish a healthy, loving and caring relationship with yourself, and when this is done you are ready to establish the same type of relationships with others and the world!

I have applied this practice many times when I was about to reach for that tempting carrot cake. First of all I would stop and leave out any type of judgment or desire to fight with the impulse. I would take a deep breath (always very important), and feel myself standing there in front of the cake, noticing my feelings, any sensations that are happening in my body and I would ask myself: "Why am I feeling like this?" "Do you have anything to tell me? Another key question that I always would ask is: "Do I really, really want it?"

I would ask this last question three times. You read correctly: three times and wait to feel the answer. I suggest the number three because you will see how the answer changes. When you are asking three times you are asking with your head, with your heart and with your soul. Trust me, it works; and even though you may get, "No, I do not want it", but still eat it, it will help you to get out of the disempowering cycle of binge eating in its own time. Simply keep applying the different practices exposed here and you will be amazed at how naturally you become free of food obsessions and a more balanced, centered and happy person.

One more thing... remember to be kind to yourself and avoid negative self-talk if you give in to food temptations and while eating it and from your heart let go of that dark energy connection which is between you. You can even say something like "It is OK... I let you go." It is OK because you are going through a process and as such you experience ups and downs and you I let go any negative, compulsive, obsessive emotion associated with food. You may tell yourself something like "I don't need you anymore" and/or, "It's time for you to go!!" Use your own words and speak from your heart. Make it a game! It really is, believe me. Have fun … don't take it too seriously because that alone makes it harder than it is.

Self-Love Exercise

Do you tell your loved ones that you love them? Do you tell them that you appreciate them? That they are important to you? Good! Now, how about if you tell yourself these things too? And how about if you tell your body, which takes you places every day and allows you to experience life the way you do, that you appreciate all which it does for you? You know, our bodies have to put up with so much abuse at times ... overeating, overworking, overexerting through exercise, fasting, etc.

It may sound ridiculous, I know because many times when I said this to friends they put on this face full of surprise and laugh. Well, I decided not to care because in the end it is I who is going to reap the rewards. So, I invite you to give yourself a hug and to send and feel love within yourself, and ignore the rest. I am not talking about becoming a full-of-yourself, arrogant type of person, an Adonis. I am simply saying that love has to start with you and end with you.

Application:

A few years ago I decided that I was going to implement this practice here and there, with no routine, just to boost my confidence my self-love. When binge eating came up in my life with such force, and after battling with it and resisting it, I decided to see it from a different perspective and apply full compassion to myself. Full compassion means no judgment, no labels, and complete acceptance. So I decided to talk to myself with love, understanding and trust, as if I was dealing with a near-and-dear-to-me trusted friend. It is funny how tolerant and caring we can be with others but so hard on ourselves, right?

Anyway, what I would do, if I found myself overeating with an anxious desire was to treat myself with tenderness and tell myself things such as "It is OK; this will pass." "I am doing my best and I can work this one out". "I am safe and this is just a temporary experience… I am letting go and it goes away." "I accept myself".

These are in no way affirmations. These are things that you say to yourself once, at any given time and then let them go.

There are plenty of opportunities to express love to oneself. Another one I often do is in the morning after taking my shower while I am still in the bathroom. If you take showers and have a mirror in the bathroom you can do it too ☺ Look at yourself in the mirror, into your eyes, hug yourself, pinch your cheeks, and tell yourself how much love and appreciation you have for your whole being. Thank the body for all it does for you. This effort is helping you regain the balance and health you want. It only takes a few seconds. It is more important the feeling, the intensity of it than the time. You do not need to make this into a structured routine... Lately I have found myself "romancing" myself spontaneously anywhere, and there is nothing that feels better than feeling and expanding in love for oneself. What can be more healing and empowering than that? What can be more inspiring?

You do not have to wait until tomorrow to do this. You do not have to wait until you attain "perfectionhood" or "sainthood". In fact, toss perfectionism and the need to be like Mother Teresa out the window! Be you and do this right now. And repeat often. No matter how "good" or "not that good" you think you are doing, remind yourself that life is a journey filled with experiences and that you are...

Doing Your Best

Yes. Every step of the way you are doing your best with the resources you have available, your motivation and desires. Did you know that... you are human too? Yes, you carry divine essence but you cannot deny your humanness–and the beauty of it.

It is important to be aware that your levels of energy, motivation, inspiration and drive vary from day to day, and that no matter how much you want to be free from old patterns and unserving emotions, they have kind of a "mind of their own". They are very resilient and stubborn and do not want to leave just like ... pooff! They like to put up a fight and defend their territory. One thing is to say: "I give you permission to go ... GO!" and other is the timing of it and how it happens. I wish it was faster, or that there was a switch to turn it off but that is not the case. I had to go through it too and so will you but the good news is that it is super-doable. It takes some time but time in one of the things that goes really fast, don't you think?

If you really want to do this you will see how in less time than you think your desire to stuff yourself with food and sweets starts to diminish and your thinking and obsessing about food starts to fade away. It is a natural process that is unique to each person and at times it is very subtle. As you start engaging in other activities that are pleasurable and meaningful to you this clinging to certain foods will lose power.

So, ask yourself if you are doing your best and keep doing it. Give your best when doing the exercises provided herein and choose to remain open to change. In short: BE you and allow the wisdom of life to fill in the details.

Application:

One of the things I have understood is that in no way am I "perfect" according to human standards and that life does not happen in a linear ascending way. I comprehended that it is OK to take three steps forward, two backwards, so on and so forth. That is simply the way it is. I had very ingrained in me the concepts of discipline, structure, willpower and force and this brought me to be hard on myself many times. Now, I am seeing myself with gentle eyes, and I have learned to be accepting and forgiving of myself. I stopped talking in negative terms about myself and I made the decision to eradicate doubt and fear from my life. I strive to see every opportunity as a chance to practice acceptance and trust, knowing that for one reason or another I am on the track that I am. I continue giving my best with the knowledge and resources I have and allow life to do the rest. This has been very liberating. Another one of the things that has helped me, and which will help you immensely to put life into a new perspective is…

Discernment

Discernment is one of the most important gifts you as a human being have at your disposal and which can bring lots of clarity and freedom. When you use discernment in a situation you reach new levels of understanding. You get deep insights, a sense of knowingness that reveals to you fresh perceptions of what is really happening, and why. Discernment is the key to reveal the truth, to get to the bottom of things and to understand oneself with no blindfolds or excuses.

Somehow it is easier to live our lives accepting what comes to us–no questions asked, seeing just the obvious and neglecting to explore what is beyond appearances, but thanks to discernment we can lift the veil and see what is really hiding behind an apparent situation and see it from a different point of view.

Application:

As I said before, overcoming binge eating is a process that has its ups and downs which means that it will take some time for you to conquer it completely. It is vital that you are aware of this fact and that you are patient and trust yourself at all times, even when you are going through a very dark moment and it seems impossible. The gift of discernment will help you, as it has helped me, to identify the reasons why you are having a strong desire for overeating in a given moment. Not all impulses to overindulge have the same motivation. For example, if you had an argument with a loved one that left you upset and you find yourself immediately reaching for a chocolate cookie, by applying discernment to the situation you will be able to see clearly that your motivation to eat that cookie comes from a negative emotion you are experiencing, and you will have the chance to choose what to do, if to go for it or perhaps breathe, let the emotion go through you and dissolve, and discover that in the end you did not need that cookie after all.

In my own experience I found that as I practised discernment, it became easier for me to identify when my desire for eating something or to overeat was due to a certain emotion I was experiencing (one I did not want to feel), and when it was just a simple desire to enjoy a little treat with no hidden agendas. On several occasions when I was feeling anxious for one reason or another, I experienced a strong impulse to run for food but by applying right away the gift of discernment, most of the time I was able to say "no" to the impulse and forget about it. The cool thing is that as quickly as it comes, it goes, no matter how strong it is. If you apply the concepts we have talked about here it goes much more easily.

Letting Go

Previously we talked about letting go of old grudges and hurts so now let's talk about letting go of something else that is pivotal: your need for binge eating. "What?" "How can you say I need this? … That is cruel!" you may be saying. Well, in my personal experience I found that even binge eating, as uncomfortable and self-destructive as it can be, it has its benefits too. You see, by eating with no control and getting yourself physically sick, exhausted and overwhelmed with negative feeling such as shame and remorse you are limiting yourself. You are holding yourself back and preventing yourself from expanding and expressing all you can be, of living your life to the fullest. You are taking away health, energy, clarity of mind, motivation, self-love and self-confidence and replacing all that with an array of non-constructive emotions and physical sensations. And the gain is? That you can hide your maximum potential, your TRUE self behind this excuse and you simply keep gliding through life surviving but not thriving.

Why? Because it is easier, more comfortable and familiar to do "nothing". Perhaps because down deep you have fear, feelings of unworthiness, doubt, or are unsure about what path to take or, "What if it is the wrong one!?" I have gone through many of these believe me, and I know perfectly what I am talking about. It may not be your case, but I invite you to take an honest, brutally honest look at yourself and ask yourself: "What benefits are binge eating giving me?" "Why am I choosing overeating?" "How does it serve me?" And then let it go!

Application:

How do you let go? Well, I am sure that you will get the answer of why you are experiencing food obsessions and the trick is that when you get your insights, do not overanalyze or try to think your way out. Instead keep the conversation with yourself (yes, I am going back to what we have discussed before), and say something like: "I let go of my need for binge eating". Say it once and let it go. Do not force anything and do not dwell on it. Later on you will find yourself saying this spontaneously once more here and there, and that is OK. As long as you do not put brain muscle into it. Because it will not do any good to you and the result will be limited. I perfectly understand that you would like to make it disappear like a magician making a rabbit evaporate but again, for most people it does not happen that way so stick with your honest desire of letting go and move to the next step which is…

Trust

Yes, trust is paramount in life! In the end you can control only a portion of your life; the rest happens no matter how much effort you are putting into it to make it happen or to avoid it happening, have you noticed?

It is normal that at moments you feel lost, lonely, or even trapped. You are not sure if what you are doing is working or not, and you wonder: "For how long will things be like this!?" My suggestion is to feel good about the things you can control and are doing to the best of your ability at the moment, and remember that the rest you have to trust. Also remember that you got to "this" place for a reason and that now that you are gaining clarity and doing your share, you have all it takes to get yourself out of it. You need YOU and only YOU in this process. All in life has its place and its time. All is appropriate. You are where you are because that is the best place for you to be in that very moment and as soon as you are ready to move to the next step the bridge will appear in front of you. Remind yourself of that, tell yourself that, and keep going with your life making the best of it every minute, because it never returns! Believe me, things do get better one step at a time.

Application:

Trust is something that has to be nurtured almost every day because our human condition finds it easier to fall into the trap of fear, drama and difficulty. I frequently remind myself of letting go what I cannot control and be proactive about what I can. A moment of big trust that I want to share with you was when I was approaching 40 kilos (88 lbs), and still had no clue of what was going on with me. My husband was extremely concerned for me, as you may imagine, and did not know what else to do. The incredible thing was that I was at peace and trusting that I was going to be fine. It was impossible for me to transmit this feeling to my husband but I hoped he would sense it somehow and that it would give him some comfort. Of course we had always been communicating openly. I knew down deep that I had to trust the process I was going through and give all of myself to it. I intuitively knew that there were more than physical things involved in it and that I had to connect with my heart, my truth, my soul, and be open to unknown outcomes. Yes, it is very important to...

Be Open

…And remain open. To be open means trust; to be closed means fear. Being open calls for a welcoming attitude towards the gifts of life, revelations and possibilities.

Being open means not engaging in a struggle with life wanting to manipulate outcomes because "you know better". Be open and keep your eyes wide open, your antenna up, because you may get signs and clues that are so fleeting that you could miss them.

An "aha!" moment, an important insight, a key contact, the perfect book, the encouraging words you need to hear, etc., may appear in front of you in the least expected way to give you some direction on what could be the next step for you to take, and if you are focusing only on what you think you want and the way you want it, a sign may come to you flashing out and still you could not see it in front of your eyes! You and I have a limited vision so, what about if we leave the details to life?

Application:

One of the things that I have been doing consciously is to remain open and attentive to receive and see life's hints. To me it is like a game, one very fun to play. I notice things that many people do not notice, and without applying brain effort I allow myself to sense the meaning of it. I believe that if I notice something meaningful it is because it is more than what it appears to be.

Serendipitous encounters, messages in billboards, personalized license plates, trees, animals, and other things, have served me as mediums to deliver a key message in a given moment.

I also know that nothing happens for no reason, or out of luck. Looking back for example, and reflecting on all I went through during these past three years, I realize more and more that every single thing, book, person, healer I met … all the dreams I had and the synchronicities I experienced had their perfect place and time in the broad scheme of things. I trusted my intuition and paid attention to what my body and heart were trying to tell me and allowed myself to be led from one thing to the next, and then to the next, and so on.

As I felt that I had obtained the tools I needed to move forward and try something else (for example a new healing method, read another book, or try other foods), life would bring to me the right person or information to get to the next level. All happened with its own rhythm and it was fascinating to me to see how life was orchestrating these opportune encounters and findings.

I was never afraid of giving things a try as I was willing to see how they would make me feel and helped me. I tried healing therapies I had never heard of before and started to see messages on car plates, billboards, magazines, songs, etc. Life, in a very natural way, was helping me to connect the dots and the more I paid attention (without being fixated on it), the more "stop signs" it would throw at me.

So, I encourage you to open yourself up to the world or possibilities and probabilities. I invite you to say, instead of "never", "why not?" You will see how the answers you are looking for start coming to you in different presentations. Take this book for instance. It is no coincidence that you found your way to it and now are reading it (lucky me ☺!).

Today I perfectly understand that I had to go through lots of stuff to be able to get to this point, and I am OK with it. I even appreciate the opportunity and the gift of life because the way I now feel about myself, my relationship with others, with food and the world is not the same thanks to it. I am embracing life with a higher sense of humor, fluidity, trust and wonder. I am accepting and loving myself in ways that I never thought possible before–and I cannot wait to see that you also experience this and all the richness that life has to offer you!

Do Something Different Every Day

One of the things that can help you to be more open is to try something different every day–and this does not have to be a big deal. I know that breaking the routine can be challenging at first because it means disruption and we tend to like the comfort zone, the familiar territory.

The good thing is that you do not have to make major changes to realize how beneficial and fun this is. You do not have to walk to your office every day, get a tattoo on your chest or dye your hair orange. You can start with small things and as you do, you will see that you start acquiring new perspectives and ideas. You start connecting with your intuition much, much easily.

So, I challenge you to do something different every day for a week at least. As I said before it can be something really simple such as calling a loved one you rarely call and expressing your love and appreciation to him or her. It can be driving home by taking a completely different route, wearing a color you have never worn before, smiling to a child you encounter, or having what you would normally have for lunch at breakfast.

Application:

In general I love variety but to tell you the truth I have found it challenging to break certain routines, especially when it had to do with food. I have carried many beliefs about food for a long time–I have to be honest… it has not been an easy task but, not impossible. Here are some of the things I have done differently – and many of them I still do:

Eat sautéd vegetables with eggs at breakfast instead of bread, pancakes or any other food made with flour. Go for a walk around the neighborhood at 11:00 pm instead of 7:00 am. Start the day by doing something I really enjoy, something fun, and then getting into work mode. Work at 4:00 am if I am not sleepy and have a nap at 5 pm if I get tired. Try ethnic recipes, herbs and spices.

See? Simple! Try it yourself for a week and see how it goes.

Be Playful, Be Silly, Laugh More!

One of the things that "grownups" avoid like a plague is to be seen as silly, or ridiculous. We do not want to feel out of place neither be censored nor criticized in any way, right? We have buried down deep the care-free, child-like spirit we all carry inside for the sake of being a serious, proper adult. I say... who cares? "Life is short!" It fades away quickly to be taken that seriously. Why not enjoy ourselves, those around us and the world a bit more? Why not have fun with the simplest things life has to offer and enjoy them with an attitude of wonder?

When I was little I was considered overly free-spirited and hard to contain. I was a girl who wanted to be out and about most of the time touching life, experiencing nature, getting wet in the rain and jumping in the puddles, climbing trees... playing all the time. My mom, who liked to control things and favored perfection and discipline, had a hard time to bring me to order, and I bet at times I made her cry... what a naughty girl! She used to take life way too seriously, most of the time, although she had a very good sense of humor... strange.

Anyhow, the day for me was way too short to do all I wanted to do. I had a source of endless energy and a hard time to concentrate and stay still in the classroom. I loved adventure and felt trapped. I wanted to be free like the wind. And free like the wind, I failed 4th grade because math did not agree with me. It was too boring. I preferred the outdoors—to play ball, to chase animals, to invent games. Anything but math! That was a year when there was not a week when I was not taken to the principal's office by my teacher due to my lack of discipline. "What are we going to do with you, Monica", they would ask out loud. And I would feel so humiliated. I did not understand what I was doing wrong.

Anyhow, after failing 4th grade I received a big and strong scolding from my mom and I spent my entire vacation studying—guess what? Math! I repeated the course and barely passed it and finally arrived to 5th grade… phew!

And that was when my life took a sharp turn I never suspected. My 5th grade teacher, Mary, ended up being "the mother of terror and discipline". She was super strict and loved to terrorize us by screaming and popping her eyes out. One of my classmates used to wet herself in front of the classroom while giving her answers. Mary probably had a very good heart, I now know, but one that held many hurts, I presume.

Mary did the "miracle". She disciplined me through terror and I became the number one student for almost the rest of school… My parents did not have to worry about my homework anymore. I started to suppress my energy and playful spirit and became a poster girl, the "favorite" of Mary! There was less nagging from my mom and more peace at home which was nice and made me feel more accepted, I guess.

I am very aware that we all need discipline and direction. We are social beings that live in a community and there is a need for boundaries, respect and commitment. Today, I can tell you that I really appreciate the sense of responsibility and discipline I learned from my mom, especially, because it has served me very well in many ways. The only thing, I feel, is that she and my dad never really understood my nature and did not know how to creatively direct me with my raw energy, how to nurture that spirit in a creative way.

The messages that stuck with me were: "You are bad". "You are trouble". "We do not love you enough IF you behave this way". "You are too much to handle", etc. I imagine that to fit in, enjoy more peace at home and school and be accepted, I controlled myself too much, without realizing that I was feeding "the rebel" within me. This rebel, one day, would jump out and say, "Now it is my time!" I never suspected that this rebellious part of me would come back with vengeance and manifest itself through my weakest point: food and more than anything my love for sweets. As an adult, not having Mom hovering around or Mary screaming at me, I was free to do whatever I pleased, including overeating all that "sweetness of life" that I greatly missed.

The funny thing is that while my eating habits started going out of control I still was very disciplined and inflexible in other areas of my life. I was very hard on me ... my worst enemy when it came to create expectations about me or judge myself.

Balance ?

I found that I ignored the full meaning of the word balance... I was more about extremes: If I worked, I had to work 16 hours a day. If I partied, I had to party until 7:00 am. If I ate, I had to eat until I dropped on the floor ballooned and feeling ill! Yes. I did not know what balance was really about and did not understand that balance was precisely what I was craving.

Application:

Life is short and it is already too serious out there don't you think? I invite you to lighten up, freshen up your life and enjoy from your heart more and more the little wonders you come across every day. Do not wait to go to a comedy to laugh or to the Grand Canyon to be marveled. Day after day life offers you many opportunities to be playful, to dare yourself to do something outrageously fun.

Be more humorous with yourself and others. Give yourself permission to do silly things, to laugh at you, just for the fun of it, just because you are here now and won't be forever and ever.

I can tell you right now that gobbling down brownies, ice cream or carrot cakes, as tasty as they are, they won't fill your heart, expand your spirit nor make you feel complete and connected with your purpose. When you have fun, when you do something that brings true joy to your heart, know that you are opening magic pathways that connect you to your spirit, to your inner innocent child, your unique creative being which knows you well and see that you are whole, lovable and perfect just the way you are! You, yes, you amigo, have it ALL inside. You do not need to get it from the bakery or ice cream parlor.

Create Something Everyday

There is a Van Gogh, a Mozart, a Shakespeare, a Caruso and there is a YOU… only one YOU! And that is a gift in itself. You are unique in all ways. You have your own traits and creative powers waiting to be tapped into and expanded. And the nice thing about it is that you do not have to study art for years or burn your eyes learning how to read notes. Very simple and mundane things are acts of creation. Every day you have opportunities to create something different, to change something, to make it look another way. If you change it, it is something new and you have been creative!

For example, if you clean and re-arrange a messy kitchen cabinet that is full of spices, that in itself is a creation. The cabinet now is looking organized; you can find your spices easily and feel great about it. If you have a silver-plated candle holder that is looking dull and polish it, in the end what do you have? a candle holder that looks like new. If you cut some flowers from your garden and make a floral arrangement for your dining table that is a creation as well. See how simple it can be to activate your creative juices?

The idea is to recognize that you are a creator and that whatever you do is a creation of yours. Every single day you have the opportunity to create something no matter how inconsequential it seems to your eyes or the eyes of others. It wasn't there before, so you created it. You have within you a unique ability to transform things. Now, how do you want to use it? Choose to create consciously, have fun with it and see where it leads you.

Application:

To make this practice a more conscious one you can do what I do: Ask yourself, "What do I want to create today?" Just ask and see what answer you get. And do not judge it, alright? Remember that it can be a new recipe, planting orchids, coloring a book, a mandala, anything.

One day you might want to create a clean house for example, which by the way will help you to see house chores with a different perspective. Another day it could be a song or a poem. The thing is that by unleashing your creative powers without expectation and judgment, you rekindle your soul and remember who you truly are down deep and what you are capable of. This will put food (sweet or salty), in a secondary place and yourself in the first and foremost place.

Own Your Power

By rekindling your soul and reaching out to your unique self you claim back your own power, your truth, your soul. Do not confuse power with manipulation, or force. One kind of power is to own your power, to be the captain of your soul, and the other kind is to use power to make others do what you want them to do for your own benefit. What I am talking about is the first kind which is a doorway you can use to embrace yourself as a human being with divine essence. In short, it is allowing your soul to shine through your humanity in whatever you do, no matter if big or small.

Control, manipulation, oppression and cruelty have nothing to do with owning your own power. When you own your own power you exude love, self-confidence and compassion. If you look around you will notice how tons of people have given away their own power allowing others and circumstances to decide for them what to experience while on this earth. Being submissive and alienated or domineering has nothing to do with being powerful. It has more to do with fear.

When you own your power, your truth, you feel at ease with life, connected with your spirit, inspired, motivated, and free. You do not have this need of changing things or people so that "you can feel better". You do not need to gobble up tons of food to feel grounded, safe, happy or in control. You know your gifts; you express them every day; you trust yourself because you know who you are: a very special human with an indivisible spirit who has it all to create the life you want. You feel full of "you" and are not afraid of it. You are from the inside out.

Application:

For a long time I thought that owning my power was about making decisions with a strong will, trying to control life, circumstances and even others to obtain certain outcomes. That power is a waste. That is misused power and yields very poor results. Also, it is very exhausting and distracting because one thinks that one is doing it the right way and that it is going to work no matter what. But in the end it is like a dog chasing its own tale hoping to catch it… It never does!

Owning your power is about being truthful with yourself. It is about acting in accordance with what brings pure joy, peace, love, wellness to your being. It is standing firm on your gifts, your uniqueness and allowing it to come through you in your daily activities.

If you do not know what bring you joy, ask yourself: "What brings me joy"? "What do I really like to do?" And start acting upon it. You will see how your true self unfolds in front of your eyes more and more as you give it permission. One of the things that can help you accomplish this is to …

Be Authentic

Yes, being authentic is the fast track to connecting with your true self, your soul. Let me ask you something: What's the best thing about you? I will tell you... That YOU are YOU, and nobody else!

Being authentic means expressing who you truly are at the soul level, and accepting every bit of yourself, luminous or dark. When this happens you do not need to fit in anymore or to fix yourself in any way because you know and appreciate that there cannot be a better version of you than that. You finally embrace your whole being and love yourself with compassion. When you choose to live an authentic life you do not need to deny or cover up your emotions with food (or anything else) because you feel connected to your true SELF, and that feels RIGHT and EMPOWERING.

Application:

One of the things that have helped me to connect with my soul and stay true to myself is my emotions. By paying attention to how I feel it is easy for me to know what resonates with my heart, and what does not. This in turn allows me to make choices based on what makes me feel at ease, truthful to myself. As I said before our emotions are one of the best tools we have because they serve us as our inner compass – if we pay attention and trust them.

Every day, like you, I am confronted with multiple choices. What to wear, what to focus on, what to buy, whom to talk to, what to say, what project to start, etc. By expressing your authentic self in each of these life situations you are being true to yourself, reaffirming who you are, and attracting to you what you really want from life.

Eating is another situation where you can practice authenticity because you can get to a point where you know that you are eating something just to enjoy it as part of the rich experience of life. That you have chosen with the free will that comes from the soul, with a pure heart, with love, and not with fear wanting to suppress a negative emotion.

You will find out that eating in moderation certain foods labeled as "bad for you" or "fattening" for example, won't have the negative effects most people associate with them and that you do not have to have the whole 12 pieces of cake at once. Isn't that good news? I think it is. This is a shift that you will naturally experience and which will make you feel so empowered compared to those times when you ate feeling anxious, embarrassed, worried, and desperate. You will see that you have moved away from a hypnotic state to your truth, your authenticity, your power, your soul. See how it works?

When I started to practise this with food I would ask myself something that you can ask yourself too: "Who wants this? … Is it me, my true self standing on my own power or, is it the fearful, hurt child inside me looking for comfort, a quick fix, love, attention?" "Is it my soul or a part of me that feels sad, confused, lonely, powerless, tired, betrayed?"

You will know; believe me, you will. You will be able to differentiate who is in command, and that is part of the discernment process we talked about earlier.

Whatever choice you make, remember to make it consciously. If you know that it was your head which chose it and the rest (heart and soul) said no but, you still gave into it, it is OK, and you know what? Enjoy it!

That is correct. Enjoy it to the maximum by being present with your cake or ice cream or whatever it is and eat it with full awareness. Taste every bite. Feel the pleasure it gives you. Notice how it makes you feel while you eat it–and after. And please, do not spoil the moment by allowing your inner critic, "that" party pooper to nag around telling you that "you are weak … a lost cause".

That is the old, false message you picked up from someone in the past when you were little (most likely) and which you are leaving behind. Yes, you are, if you have decided to do it with your heart and are doing your very best. It is a normal part of the process to slip back into the unwanted habits once in a while (be careful this does not become an excuse).

One day, soon enough, you will be able to choose what your heart and soul tells you and you will clearly see that there was no need to force or to discipline yourself. That complete awareness plus other simple practices was what you needed.

By trusting the process and trusting yourself you will be able not only to conquer binge eating but to enjoy whatever food you like with no negative preconceptions or ill effects because you will do it under the umbrella of BALANCE. Choosing and living a more balanced way will becomes second nature to you.

This change will come from the inside, not from the outside. It will stem from your sense of self-love, self-worthiness, self-acceptance and self-confidence.

It will take some time – and that is different for each person. Personally it took me more than a year and it was something gradual. At first I was able to stop eating sweets for a while but after three months or so and when I started feeling that the cleansing of the Candida overgrowth was taking effect, cravings came back and stronger than ever. Some would argue that it was the Candida trying to get food to survive and yes, perhaps that was part of it but not all, neither the most important part of the puzzle. Candida was the perfect masquerade for all the rest that I had to experience to finally come out of the trance, the hypnotic state in which I was. I had adopted these hypnotic, erroneous ideas and beliefs about me and life, and it was time to unload them.

Some of the things that I used to crave with an incredible sense of urgency included chocolate macaroons and croissants. I confess that many times I gave in, and at the beginning I felt guilty, hopeless and doubtful. I thought that I was not going to be able to do it. But as I progressed and stuck with the simple practices I am sharing with you I started to feel that the anxiety and sense of urgency to binge was melting away, and gradually I had more and more days when I could simple say "no". Then I noticed that when I said yes I could have a much smaller portion and stop! Later I realized that this inner sense of urgency to eat right away was done. So, be patient with yourself. Again, if there is something that goes by (very quickly), it is time. One day and not that long from now, you will feel completely different about food (and yourself), and the best of all is that you will be able to savor and enjoy everything, literally everything, you want to eat. It may be too that your taste and preferences change, but those days when you decide to enjoy a piece of birthday cake, you will be able to do it, choosing from a place of inner power and contentment … and your body will be able to process it, no problem. As I said, at times I thought this was impossible because the path seemed pitch dark but I can tell you now, it is not impossible at all!

Shake The Body, Baby!

Movement is paramount when it comes to leading a more balanced life. I personally do not advocate strenuous exercise but, it is up to you to decide how you want to shake that body of yours. Similar to breathing, moving the body helps you to shake off trapped energies that are not serving you anymore and get them moving. It also helps to release hormone-like substances called endorphins, which make you feel more content and relaxed. No matter how busy you are every day I highly recommend you to set apart at least five minutes (which is nothing) to move the body in a way that is enjoyable to you.

Application:

Some of the exercises I like to do and which you may want to consider doing include: yoga, stretching and dancing. I love dancing. I think it is very fun. I like to dance Latin music, pop and sometimes even rock, depending on the mood. Many times I don't worry about the rhythm or the technique. I just close my eyes and follow what my body tells me to do. This can be a meditation in itself, did you know? If you immerse yourself into the music and move as you please being very present, then you have created an instant active meditation. Meditation does not have to be still or silent; actually anything you do with full awareness can be considered a meditation, even doing laundry!

Walking is another activity I like and do often. My husband calls me "Forrest Gump" because I can walk and walk and walk. I encourage you to take some time to go out for a walk and enjoy yourself in the outdoors. Use this time to let go of your active mind, feel your body taking each step, observe your surroundings, hear the sounds and feel the breeze. If some days you can do it only for five minutes, this is OK. Try to do it for ten minutes at least and choose different routes (this also helps to expand your awareness and intuition).

Add More LUV!

I am aware that change is something not that easy for most of us and when it means drastic change we resist it even more. My own healing journey during these last three years showed me that by taking small, achievable steps, and making it fun, the process of change kind of happens by itself, in a pleasant and natural way. They say: "What you resist persists". And it is very true.

That is why after trying so many therapies and techniques I decided to return to the basics and make things simple and enjoyable. And that is exactly the main message I want to convey in this book. **Go for the simple and fun!**

Brain power, rigidness and hard discipline, I found, is not that effective and you get the risk of dropping out in the middle of the process. Instead, steady, practical, doable and enjoyable steps are what it takes to make vital, deep rooted changes in your life. I am a proof of it. If I have been able to do it you can do it too!

Why struggle your way to balance, inner peace and happiness if it can be done with grace, simplicity and even joy?

All it takes is to say YES and continue doing so. Yes to love, yes to life, yes to you, dear friend, you, you, the precious you.

By adding a bit more of love every day into your life you naturally reconnect with your soul and heart and in less time that you can imagine, you start experiencing important shifts that make you feel empowered and joyful from the inside out.

Simple practices like those I have outlined for you here can make it easier for you to transition from binge eating to life loving–from food obsession to life creation, from self-constriction to self-expansion.

Little by little, adding more LUV into your life will help you to tear down your guards (conscious or unconscious) and melt away old emotions and unserving energies that are blocking your way and preventing you from experiencing a fulfilling life, a life that is free of worthless conditionings and fears.

You will realize that adding more LUV into your live does not mean eating pies, cookies and ice cream with no boundaries. Even if you are going through a phase where you are allowing yourself to eat whatever you want with full awareness and presence, be careful not to fall into the extreme permissive mode. Be always vigilant to know who is in command and notice if you are making excuses for not moving forward.

Adding LUV goes way beyond food, even though many of us have received demonstrations of love and care through food since we were tiny. It means engaging in other activities meaningful to you; activities that make your heart sing, that leave you with a happy aftertaste, not guilt, remorse or shame.

Every day you can add more LUVVV to your life by doing simple things such as deep breathing, going for a walk, talking to a close friend, taking a bubble bath, receiving a massage, lighting a scented candle, listening to your favorite music, surprising a loved one with a small gift, reading a fun book, watching a movie, dancing in your kitchen while cooking, etc. Every day there are plenty of opportunities to add LUVVV to your life. What do you enjoy doing? SO, go ahead and do it then!

Application

This very moment, while I am writing to you, I am sitting on the shore of Lake Ontario, working on a picnic table while listening to the waves crashing onto the beach. Yes, today the lake is quite active... it feels as if I were by the ocean! The breeze is pleasantly warm and is moving gently caressing my skin and my hair. The temperature is about 29 C (84 F) and the sun is shining with splendor, reflecting its rays on the water and making some waves look like clusters of diamonds. A day like this feels like heaven to me. By choosing to be here, now, I am adding luv into my life in a way that my whole being enjoys beyond words. I could be working in my home office, or at the library, for example. But that would be the old me, that one that favored more discipline and structure. Those days are gone. Who said that you cannot mix pleasure with work? What can be more inspiring and motivating than doing what you have set your mind to do in an environment that lifts your spirit?

Other things that I like to do to add more luv into my life include writing, dancing, acting and swimming. I enjoy impromptu dancing or unplanned acting, as well as filling up the bathtub and splashing like a little girl.

Fire Food & Other Vampires

Firing food and other vampires is an important step to take while you go about practising the different ways discussed in this book. It is key that you identify energy vampires in your life and realize their impact so that you can take appropriate and firm action! Energy vampires are very real... I have experienced them in different aromas, shapes and forms. They suck your energy out and leave you behind feeling half you: exhausted, sad, irritable, apathetic, etc.

Food can be one of them. Food has the potential to energize you, inspire you, connect you with your greatness, or drain you and make you feel all sorts of emotions such as boredom, apathy, blame, guilt and sadness. Foods loaded with sugar and unhealthy fats for example, if eaten too often and in big portions, cause blood sugar spikes making you feel energized at first but then sluggish and moody. Yes, you may feel "on top of the world" for a few minutes while you savor every bite of that chocolate cheesecake and while your body takes the sugar in, but then, after the sugar rush is gone, what is the aftermath? Let me tell you by my own experience: bloating, gas, sluggishness, crankiness, irritability, feelings of emptiness, indifference, guilt, unworthiness, and more. Not a nice picture at all.

Food can have a strong numbing effect. By making yourself feel sick and tired, with no motivation whatsoever, you are providing yourself the perfect excuse to avoid looking at important issues within you that should be dealt with so you can move to higher levels of consciousness and enjoy all that life has to offer.

Among those issues are common disempowering, false beliefs such as unworthiness, incompleteness, imperfection, lack of success, unintelligence, too fat, too short, too boring, etc. I know firsthand that it is much easier to maintain the status quo than to provoke change. Looking at oneself with a critical, objective eye is not that fun at times. But, if you do not do it, nobody will. And you won't be able to experience the richness of life. You did not come to this earth to suffer. You came to expand your wings and have a blast doing what is important and joyful to you. So… it is your call.

Do you really want to change?

What do you want to do?

How do you want to live your life? on your own terms? on the terms dictated by others and food?

By overeating certain foods that you know (yes you do), have a negative impact on your health and the way you feel you are giving away tremendous power. You are relinquishing your own and your rights and gifts to create the life you want for yourself from the core of your being, your eternal soul.

Food can be a wonderful and delicious medium to sustain our energies and enhance our health and vitality, but it also can be used as a smoke screen to hide our true selves from ghosts and dragons that in the end do not exist! How do I know? Because I have faced them right in the eye, and after much inquiring they have told me that they resulted from past experiences and repetitive conditionings and were just trying to "protect me".

They sprouted from the very same fears and false beliefs our parents, grandparents, teachers, and different authority figures had. They did not know better, but you dear friend, you do now.

You are here reading this because you have been looking for answers, for other alternatives, for simplicity, for light-heartedness. You know that there must be another way, and you want to get to it and you want to wake up and get going with your life with no smoke screens, empowered and free to choose what you TRULY want in your heart – not with what you think you want or the fearful inner child in you is making you believe you want.

I say: Fire the food vampires! Tell each food you are overeating and obsessing over that it is fired! That it can go away and only come back in a balanced way. I know–silly? Do it anyway. You will see how attentive they are to your heartfelt commands.

Now, there are other vampires lurking around waiting to latch on and suck your energy, and whose attack can lead you easily to crave certain comfort foods – if you are not alert and are not standing on your power. These vampires have legs and arms and big mouths. They are people. They do not wear black capes nor have large teeth. They have a thirst, not for blood but for an energy boost and they want to get it from someone else... you. They have a tendency to live a life of drama and victimhood. Supposedly they can make your life miserable but the truth is that it is not about them, but you. You have the power to say no. You have the power to put boundaries and make them respect them. Or, you can allow these people to suck your energy out. These energy vampires can be found among family members or coworkers. No matter "who" they are, when you relinquish your inner power to them, you are opening your veins allowing an instant transfusion of energy that leaves you drained, depleted, moody, angry, and much more.

I have experienced it many times but now that I'm very aware of it, anytime I encounter one, I make a conscious decision to not fall into their game. I decide to keep at bay their negative energy charge that they want to exchange for my own precious energy.

I realize that I'm not responsible for anyone's happiness or misery, no matter how much I care for them. I am a grown up person so are they, so are you. Allowing people to steal your energy and live off you is not good for anybody... It is not healthy for you or for them, and you know why? Because personal growth results from taking responsibility. From accepting and dealing with your own stuff, the geography of your life which may include all kinds of mountains, valleys, deserts, rivers, icebergs, forests and dark caves.

If you are allowing someone to be your energy vampire it is time to realize it and let him or her go. Notice that if after coming across this person you feel an urge to eat and binge. Notice how you think about food and which type of foods you want to eat right after. Notice your breathing pattern too. You may find out that you are gasping for some air, that you are becoming anxious. If you become aware of this you will be on the fast track to making the right choices for you, to living your life for yourself and choosing what empowers you and connects you with your true self. Trust me, I've been there.

You see... you don't have to please every single person that comes to you. That would be an impossible task to accomplish anyway. You do not have to say yes to every single favor asked of you. You don't have to compromise your tranquility and freedom simply because you have a big, loving heart. It is OK to put boundaries. It is more than

OK to say NO. It is fine to do what you really, really feel like doing in a given moment. Trust yourself and you will see how much lighter you feel. You will have more energy to focus on what is important to you. You will feel a sense of self-respect. You will have more clarity. Your zest for life will increase as well as a general sense of well-being. This is one of the key things that will help you accomplish your heart's desires—and that includes stopping food binging and obsessing over those sweet treats and baked goodies.

It is a personal choice. And the great thing about this is that when you take responsibility others cannot help but notice, so that your actions become an inspiration to those observing closely. You, my friend, are an inspiration… act like one!

Application:

I have to admit that I struggled with firing food. Being a strong-willed person wanting to "be the boss" it was difficult to me to let go and say to myself, "I do not HAVE to have that food now", because at the same time another, strong part of me was telling me, "have it… you are the boss!" I succumbed many times to the "boss" story and did as I pleased but not without consequences.

The consequences included feelings of emptiness, anxiety, fatigue, apathy, insomnia, constipation, and even muscle and joint pain. I knew that an excessive amount of sugar and flour was draining me and keeping me in a zone far away from my true self, and still I was doing it because I wanted it that way, I had to have the reins, you see?

It would take me three to five days to regain my vitality and motivation and it wouldn't be long until the "boss" appeared again and once more the cycle would begin. But one day I understood that I was the boss, not food. Food was acting like an energy vampire that could care less about me. Really! So I chose to fire it, and said it loud and clear.

Simultaneously, I decided to add more luv into my life big time! I embarked into different projects and started doing things that I enjoyed, constantly reminding myself, "who" the real boss was. I chose life instead of a slow, "bite by bite" death. Putting all that food in my body was killing me softly (like the song). It was not only making me sick but it was literally killing any possibility to express my soul on this earth and enjoy the abundance of life, and for what? for a bar of chocolate? "Is that really worth it?" I thought, "No way!"

Another example... For years I took on other people's trials and tribulations. I felt that I was a savior of sorts, that by taking on my friends' and relatives' problems, I was going to spare them aggravation and suffering until one day I had an epiphany and realized that what I was doing was no favor to any of us. I was volunteering myself to being crucified. I was losing my North, my purpose, my precious energy and even health. I decided then to let them be, to let them have their own experiences, to hit their own walls repeatedly if necessary, to have full compassion. I decided to be there with them, not for them. I was not going to be there to make their homework or carry their burdens (along with mine) simply because I have a strong back and a big capacity for love. No. No more I told myself. And I started to choose ME first, and do it without judgment, without feeling selfish, bad or sad for them or myself, because in the end each of us has his own life and has to have his own experiences, even if they cause bruises.

It wasn't easy to let go and trust life's course. But again, the simple practices I applied to overcoming overeating helped me to let go of these walking vampires.

It was my choice… it is your choice … like everything else!

Conclusion

"Everything happens for a reason," they say. I truly believe it. And my recent health experience was no exception. As much as I would have loved to skip it, looking back I can see the multiple gifts contained in the maze of what I went through for three years: food allergies, food intolerances, extreme weight loss, exhaustion, complete lack of motivation, anxiety and panic attacks, muscles, joints, bones pain, eye pain, deep sadness, memory loss, fogginess, irritability, insomnia, hair loss, no menses for over a year, and other things.

After all these experiences and now sitting on the fence looking at a much greener pasture, I comprehend how strong the body and human spirit can be, and how we can find the way out of dark situations if we are willing to do it, trust and do the work.

This has not been the first time I have been sick but it has been the longest. In the past, for example, I had an incapacitating lower back pain for a whole year. I think that life (and the soul) gives us several opportunities to deal with unresolved issues and our body serves as a medium to communicate this to us.

I think that a big percentage of what happens within our body is a reflection of what is going inside us. And if you want to know why I say this, watch "Biology of Perception" a presentation on YouTube by Bruce Lipton, a very reputable scientist.

In a nutshell, here is a brief summary of what I have learned with this life experience:

- It all starts and ends with me. It is not about others or outside circumstances or people making me to do things. I know that I have the power of choice and if I execute this power, life responds and brings back to me whatever matches what I am putting out there. It's like a boomerang.

- **I have to be willing to change.** It was up to me to cut the vicious cycle of binge eating and overindulging in sweets and other foods. It was up to me to listen to my body, to give myself permission to let go those old trapped energies, to follow my intuition and my heart, not my head and my old ways of being.

- I do better with no expectations. Wow! This was a difficult lesson for me to learn, and I still have to remind myself of it once in a while when I feel tempted to apply some brain power to a situation or fear wants to show up again. No expectations has meant to me to do my best according to what feels right in my heart and let the outcome unfold in its own time and form. In the beginning, for example, I had this expectation of how my healing should be and by when I should be free of food obsession and so on. Finally I got it! I could cut myself open to release all this clogging stuff but it was not only up to me... I had to allow the process to follow its own natural path and trust that the old ingrained unserving energies would go away when it was appropriate. I made peace with it and embraced the process with no expectation.

- Letting go is freeing. Letting go has brought more peace and balance into my life. I cried my eyes out when I decided to let go of old hurts, old energies and ways of being ... I think we were like "lovers" and we had such a close relationship that it was hard to part ways. Letting go has been freeing and refreshing. My letting go has also meant freeing myself of attachments. **By the way, letting go does not mean doing nothing and allowing life or others to decide for me or see what happens.** Letting go means making a conscious decision and not being attached to the outcome: the when, the how, the who, with whom, etc. Letting go, to me, has also involved other people. Letting them experience life in the way they want to, even if that means eating the whole cake while sitting next to me! The fact that they want to overindulge and hide themselves with food does not mean that I have to do it too.

- Trust. Trust plays a key role in the equation of life and in the act of letting go. Trust includes trust in yourself no matter how lost you think you are. Trust in the wisdom of your body no matter how ill, fat, slim or weak it is. Trust in life, period. Because you are life!

- Avoid labels. We humans love labeling. We have to put a label to everything and that includes ourselves, otherwise it is like things do not exist! We use words such as dumb, ugly, unqualified, fat, not very smart, slow, tall, short, uneducated, lucky, unlucky, beautiful, etc. We also use labels to describe us according to the conditions we are experiencing. For example: arthritic, diabetic, and alcoholic. Who says that that is what we really are? That is simply a situation we may be experiencing in a given moment, but that does not define us. I finally understood having an "intense" experience with food does not make me a "foodaholic". No. I have the power to let go of the intensity and enjoy any food (even a feast if I like to), and still remain grounded and balanced. I do not have to fall again into compulsive eating, IF I do not choose it. I can stay in my true power, be true to my soul and at the same time enjoy life with all the experiences it has to offer, why not?

- The more authentic I am and the more luv I add into my life the more enjoyable my experience of life is, and the more real it feels. At times when it seemed impossible for me to stop devouring those croissants or chocolates, I opted for adding more luv at the same time. I figured: "If I add more luv into my life more love will flow through me infusing me with positive feelings and the feelings of possibilities, therefore those outdated energies that do not serve me anymore, and which I have agreed to release, will realize that there is no place for them in me anymore". Yes, that's what I did and it worked. I started to enjoy more the outdoors, dance more, sing more, create new work projects, etc. I started to play with life and create situations that I would look forward to. I noticed that the more I engaged in these things the less my interest in food was. I understood that every moment, every step of the way I had a choice: I could choose LIFE or I choose to die slowly with the belly full of food.

- No more struggle, discipline, structure, and force. I cut the cords and experimented with simpler ways to reconnect with myself and release what was inside me looking for resolution. I did too much of many disciplines and it became a chore. I was starting to feel that if I did not do "this" or "that" I was not going to make it, to heal, to feel free. I decided to throw away so many rules about food, diets and toss the labels too: "good", "bad", "healthy" and so on. I opted for something much simpler... trust my body and my heart. I used to think that if I were to follow my body's desires I would end up eating all those over-processed foods low in nutritional value, high in artery-blocking fats and the quick fix, sugar. But I found that by doing the easy-to-do practices I have shared with you I naturally cruised towards balance and life more and more.

- There is plenty of everything, for everyone, including me! And that I do not have to chase it or have it all at once because life is abundant in many ways and will continue to be. There is plenty of time to do what I want to do, plenty of food and flavors to enjoy, plenty of opportunities, money, friends and experiences to have. If I do not have a piece of cake today that does not mean that I cannot have it another day. I understood that by not eating that cake right at the moment when my inner, fearful or hurt inner child was telling me to, I was not missing out on anything special or I was not being left out of the fun. I was simply choosing from a place of balance, from my true self. I was opting to experience a different thing that could be as simple as not having it.

- Like most humans, I tend to forget rapidly. Every time I succumbed to a fest of sweets and/or other treats I was going for the instant pleasure and of course did not care about the consequences. I was feeling good at that moment and I already had forgotten how I was going to feel later on: sick, in pain, emotionally disturbed, etc. I realized how convenient it was at times to "forget" and lie to myself for the sake of a piece of brownie!

- Enjoy the ups and downs of the experience. Deep sadness does not kill! I learned that I can go to the depths of dark emotions if necessary, embrace them and come back to the surface stronger and more balanced than ever. I cried a lot but laughed at me a lot too and marveled at my capacity to feel.

- Breathe, breathe and breathe deeply. This is something that I apply as much as I can and will continue doing until my last breath. I noticed how deep breathing speeded up the healing and rebalancing process for me, and helped me many times to stay away from falling into the vicious cycle of overeating.

- Self-talk rocks! Talking to myself helped me to cruise through this adventure with more ease and even fun. It showed me how responsive my being can be to what I communicate to it no matter if it is the body, mind or spirit. Self-talk accelerated my healing process and showed me that the most important relationship I can have is with myself and the best friend I can have is my own self. That I can be a powerful ally of myself and that it can be very fun to sit down with myself and have an intimate conversation while sipping tea ☺. I also noticed that, most of the time, things I was telling another person, I was actually telling to myself. That what I was expressing was something I needed to hear. So I became attentive to what I was telling others to recognize the part of it that had to do with me. This helped me to reinforce things and get new understandings.

OK. In a smaller nutshell ;) it all boils down to very simple things:

Wanting to change, giving yourself permission to let go of the old beliefs, emotions and limitations, accepting yourself completely (dark and luminous sides), and loving yourself with compassion, knowing that you are human but that you have divine essence also; therefore, you are and can be much more than what you see in the mirror every day!

Now, wanting to change and getting the results you want are two different things. We talked about this, remember? Unfortunately (or fortunately), there is no timetable for this process of attaining balance, and each person goes through it in a different way. This is vital to keep in mind so you do not get overly frustrated and give up. **It takes time, and it is OK!** You are not racing against anybody and do not have to prove anything anymore to anyone. This is about you and what you want to do with your life, so forget about others. If you get off track, remember that you always have the power of choice at each turn. You get off track… OK, get on track again, that's all! One day, without fretting much about it and thanks to practising simple things and the steps provided in this book, you will find yourself walking the middle road more often than not.

So, I invite you to take your own hand and start this journey with a deep breath and a big smile in your heart. Put one foot forward; start moving and choosing consciously. You will see that the path is friendlier than you ever imagined because you already have inside ALL you need to transform it into whatever you want it to be. You are an awesome divine human being, so show it to the world!

Appendix

Health Mystery... What Is Going On With Me?

They say that a journey starts with the first step and I am about to take "another" first step today. This will be the beginning of a tale about my own journey to health in the hope that it may inspire others to look carefully at their own situations not just from a bio-chemical viewpoint but also emotional and spiritual. We are multi-faceted beings who need to take care of the whole being. May my experiences help you with your own journey. Many of the procedures I followed were steps that each had its purpose despite not being continued for a long period. Each one led me to new insights and to the next step. The choice to go to a new one was a very personally motivated decision, not always consciously directed. The path may seem to you sporadic and not "logical" but I firmly believe I needed to follow them this way for me. Your journey may be completely different. The inspiration will be in the fact that all happened as it should.

It All Started In The Stomach

This chapter of my life started about three years ago although in reality it had started much earlier than that. The thing is that the change was so subtle that I hadn't noticed it (or perhaps I wasn't ready to notice), until it became an obvious health challenge! I started to have hormonal and digestive issues, something that had never been a problem before.

33 Pounds Gone!

Suddenly I was not digesting grains, then meat and poultry, then eggs–you name it! It came to a point where even water was too much for me. I was experiencing heartburn after drinking water! This made me buy the very first supplement for what would become an interesting healing and releasing journey. It was a liquid supplement that alkalized the water. I paid a small fortune for some mineral drops. But they helped to some extent.

I wasn't eating that much so of course I started to lose weight like a skydiver in free fall. I lost 20 pounds (about 10 kilos) in about a year and then lost another 13 pounds within the next 6 months. I am 5.7 feet.

The funny thing is that what I was eating was very healthy. I'd been learning about nutrition and natural health for almost 15 years so I thought I knew how to eat in a healthy way.

Handfuls Of Hair Gone

My hair started to fall out in handfuls. I was scared to wash my hair. I've always had tons, so much so that my mom used to have trouble managing it when I was little. I didn't care. Actually, I liked it "afro ". She obviously didn't and we had our intense moments over it.

Up until the summer of 2007 I had enjoyed long, thick, curly, strong hair but very quickly it was going down the drain. I started cutting it shorter and shorter because it was too tiring for me to wash.

I checked my thyroid (I had other typical symptoms of it being low), but the doctor said that it was fine. I did the basal temperature test at home and found that it was a bit under the normal range.

No Energy … Lots Of Contemplation

My energy levels started to drop and fast! I had none, not even to do even the simplest and easiest things such as washing the dishes. Many times I'd let them pile up for my husband to take care of in the evening. My arms were hurting a lot so lifting and holding things was challenging. It was as if I had fibromyalgia. But I never thought I had that.

For days and days I'd feel like doing very little, almost nothing. The only thing I wanted to do was to sit down on the couch and meditate. During summer I used to drive to the lake, 8 minutes from home, and sit down by the water or lie on the grass to energize myself. It was a phase filled with contemplation.

At night I was so exhausted that many times my husband had to help me undress and put my pajamas on. — Wow. Looking back in my mind at those days seems like a bad dream!

Heavy Duty Cramps & Knees Locking Up

I started to experience strong cramps at night and sometimes during the day. I especially remember one that left me with a sore calf muscle for two weeks. I was walking with my friend Gail in Ft. Lauderdale. We were attending a seminar and had gone out to eat something. Suddenly it hit me and I thought I was going to pass out because of the incredible pain.

People stopped and asked if they could do something. I signaled "no". What I did do was to put in practice what I had learned from Caroline and Eckhart Tolle from the sessions and books I had been reading. More about that later.

Another thing that started to happen was that my knees, specially the right one would lock up at night or while sitting at the table.

One time my husband had to pull the couch close to the dining table and helped me to lie down on it with my leg bent. I stayed there for an hour or so, feeling the sensation and sending it energy–something I'd been learning lately.

After an hour I was able to stretch the leg, get up and go to sleep. This happened many times and I remember that during last episode, after three hours of no mobility, I finally thought of applying a hot and humid towel to the area, which helped me to regain movement much faster.

Moments like this made me appreciate much more the freedom of movement and the gift of health. It's not that I'd been taking my health for granted. I've always been appreciative of what I have but I was going through a different set of circumstances that I'd never experienced before.

Asleep? Or, Out Of Body!

At night I was so exhausted that falling asleep was not that bad but for more than a year I woke up many times during the night. It became the norm for me and somehow I was able to "function" next day. I would toss and toss, meditate, visualize, do deep "belly" breathing, hum, count sheep or clouds–nothing worked!

A couple of times I had very vivid, unusual experiences. I felt that I was out of my body and in one of these sessions, I would feel brave enough to look at myself and see me lying on the bed in my pajamas! Was it real? Some would say "no way!" To me, however, it was more real than the fingers typing this!

Ice Cubes In Hands & Feet

One of the things that I found bothersome was that I was cold all the time. My feet and hands were normally frozen and this was not just in winter time when I had to wear 3 layers of clothes to keep my body warm. Since I had lost all that weight I could afford wearing all those layers and not look too thin. My bony body was not that obvious under the layers which included thermal underwear pants, corduroys, turtlenecks, sweaters, sometimes a jacket and of course always a long puffy coat.

From Size 5-6 To Size 12 Junior

At the beginning of this three year "unique episode" I was wearing size 5-6. At my lowest point in terms of size, energy and zest for life I was size 12 junior! I looked like a stick with fortunately still lots of hair despite that it was falling like crazy.

I remember when my niece came from abroad to study English in the summer of 2009, her eyes welled up but as she was about to cry, I stopped her in her tracks with a "No, no, no. There's nothing to cry about. I'm well and I'm getting better".

I had the confidence and she could see it, I guess. I knew all was temporary and that this experience would also be so one day soon.

Zero Motivation, Mixed Emotions & Lost Soul

For months and months my motivation was extremely low. My excitement for life was gone. My mood would change in the snap of a finger and my soul I guess was wandering around trying to re-connect with me somehow. At one point I started to feel as if I was drying up inside. It felt that my inner flame was extinguishing rapidly.

Limited Thinking Process, Poor Memory & Lack Of Focus

I started to notice that my thinking was not too clear, that I was forgetting many things and couldn't concentrate as easily anymore. At times it was even funny to notice all the silly things I was doing! Placing things where they didn't belong for example was common.

Thank goodness I've always tried to see the glass half full and most of the time I was able to laugh at myself. One thing I tried to do as much as possible was to keep a good sense of humor during this whole process. But on some occasions the strength of my emotions and irritability ruled the moment. And I allowed this too. I knew it was part of the "deal" and that I had to be patient and compassionate with myself. I made sure to let those around me know about this so they could understand a spontaneous burst into tears, because…

Spontaneous Crying

Yes, a flood of spontaneous tears could roll down at any moment. Many times while having dinner for example, the flash of a childhood memory would come to me and I'd start crying. I had so many good cries–heartfelt cries, the kind that empty the vessel.

Again, I recognized and accepted that this was all part of a deep healing process that was taking place. There were many things repressed inside me that were straining to go afloat and I needed to be aware to allow their release.

Reading & Absorbing Self Help Info

While all this was happening, I was reading as much as I could to understand myself better and make the most out of this process. My eyes were hurting and were tired so I couldn't read as often as I wanted to but, the good thing was that Oprah was running her famous "Soul Series" so I was able to listen to her incredible interviews on the computer.

Eckhart Tolle and Osho were among my favorite authors. I also discovered Doreen Virtue and a website called www.worldpuja.com which was very helpful and inspiring. I read other enlightening books that I'll tell you about later.

My Body Is Speaking!

At the beginning, I thought there was just something wrong with my body. Maybe I'm sensitive to some foods. Maybe I have a nutrient imbalance, or toxins. Who knows? And yes, that was part of the whole picture but not all nor do I think the most important.

Of course my husband was very worried about my weight and all the symptoms I had. By February 2009 I was looking like a malnourished third world child, and this isn't an exaggeration. I was about size 12 junior and I could count my ribs as could anyone who gave me a hug. But…

I Was Not A Victim

You may be wondering if at this point I felt like a victim. Why me, God!??

Not really. I never considered myself a victim nor allowed anyone to treat me like one. I knew in my core being that there was something special about this process even though sometimes it was far from fun or pleasant at all.

There was something profound taking place and I wanted to find out what it was!!

Now, looking back I also realize that perhaps I also wanted to test myself… I don't know, maybe. Maybe I had this subconscious desire to see how far I could take this – and be a witness to my own healing process.

I Want To See My Dragons & Monsters

The weaker I got (and lighter), the more interested I became in my own self. My emotions, unsolved issues, fears, insecurities, life perceptions, life interpretations, all that stuff we are made of, had to have the clues I was looking for or so I thought.

I was feeling the process and at the same time using myself as an "experiment".

In my own lab (my physical body), I was experiencing layer by layer what was bottled up in my soul and emotional being and I was trying to understand it.

I was more concerned, but not even that, perhaps I could say, more "curious" about those issues, the dragons and monsters that were hiding in the caverns of my being perhaps for years, decades!

Perhaps some of you might think that I was a bit (or a lot) cuckoo–crazy for having chosen to live this life experience the way I was. In short, I was trusting myself and trying to re-connect with that part of me that in the past had been so confidant and strong, my own intuition, my soul.

"Did I Go To The Doctor?"

Oh yes! My husband was very concerned and to rule everything out I went to see my family doctor. I was weighing about 48 kilos (96 pounds) when I went to his office. He ordered all the exams and tests possible:

- Blood test
- Urine test
- Test for parasites
- MRI
- CT Scan
- Ultrasound
- X-rays

Nothing! Nothing showed up. All was "good". Of course all was good! Life and soul issues don't show up in X-rays! I was going through a metamorphosis. I was like a snake changing its skin but in a way that couldn't be detected with traditional machines and tests.

My Own Discoveries

I have a very inquisitive and curious mind (I think I got that from my father who was an MD), and that makes me an avid reader and researcher. At this point in my life I had accumulated tons of info on food and nutrition; so, according to what I knew and was feeling in my body, I started to change my diet. I was eating less meat in general, juicing like crazy and eating smaller portions. I was eating more nuts and raw foods.

I wasn't really expecting anything major from the medical tests, although I have to confess that a part of my mind, the little human self that likes to worry and be fatalistic at times wondered about cancer for example. But I didn't feel there was anything really out of whack with my body that I couldn't handle. The thing I didn't consider was that it would take me a while to get to the bottom of all this BUT, it had to be this way, I now know.

And now, here are the actual steps I took as I wandered from one inspired "aha" to the next.

Connecting The Dots For True Healing And Transformation

As I said earlier in Part I, this phase of my life started about three years ago, although I know that I had been carrying the seeds for it for a long, long time.

What I'm going to share with you now are all the things I did to get back on track to regain my health, vitality and love for life.

I had to do this by myself because there was no other way. It took a while for me to figure it out but, I don't regret any decision I made along the journey because all of what happened had its own time and its own place in the whole scheme of things.

All helped me in one way or another and enriched my experience of life, and ultimately my whole being, the person I've become – and still am becoming every day.

I believe for me it was written in the stars that I had to go through this path somehow, and I did!

Nobody could have done the homework for me because it was about more than losing my health for a while. It was about transformation–clearing lots of mental and emotional baggage, learning new ways of being, re-connecting with myself and being re-born… Let me start with the first step I took in this exciting, healing journey!

Painful "Chinese" Reflexology

During the summer of 2007 I went to see a Chinese doctor, also a reflexologist, Li Zu Dan, because I was feeling tired, my lower back was hurting and I was experiencing digestive and hormonal issues.

This doctor had graduated as an MD in Beijing and was a certified reflexologist here in Canada. A Korean friend told me about him and we went together to my first appointment. I only saw him for three months because his office was about 50 minutes from my home, so it wasn't very convenient.

He had invented a tool, like a wooden stick, which he used instead of his hands to put pressure on those sore points on the bottom of the feet. These points indicate that energy is blocked in some part of the body.

He would make me scream–literally. I would squirm almost non-stop in that chair for 30 minutes. It was very painful. One of my nieces can testify to this because I took her a few times. He adjusted my back giving me great results. My energy levels increased, digestion improved, the lower back pain was going away and also my hormones seemed to be balancing out. Nonetheless, because it was far and after each treatment I was almost too tired to drive back, I stopped this treatment and continued my search.

Bio-Energy Therapy & Karmic DNA

Around the same time I was seeing doctor Li, I started to work with Rose Saroyan, a Bio-Energy therapist certified in Karmic DNA therapy. Another friend told me about Rose and how amazing her sessions were. She said that she used a very unique method that only very few people knew to help people understand their life's purpose, what made them tick, their big and small challenges and possible causes of disease, etc.

I worked with Rose during the whole summer. She helped me gain clarity and confirm many things that I'd been pondering for a long while. She provided me with remarkable insights about myself and my relationship with others and the world, some of which would come to me like flashes of insight.

My experience with Rose was very revealing and exhilarating too. She helped me to put things together, to understand why I felt and behaved the way I did. I began to see things in regards to my life, my gifts and challenges, my life's purpose, my relationship with others, my behavior patterns, etc., in a new light. These continue to come to me even now.

She also taught me about an amazing Hawaiian practice called Ho'oponopono which served me very well. It is an ancient Hawaiian code and means of forgiveness to make amends with the people with whom you have a relationship as well as with your ancestors. Its main purpose is to forgive others as well as yourself of any wrongdoing towards them whether intentional or not. Today Dr. Hew Len is one of its main promoters.

Health & Healing Workshops

During the following months I attended several workshops on nutrition and health as well as alternative and complementary medicine. I was hunting for answers. The local Whole Foods supermarket hosted some good ones where I met two people that helped me a lot along the way. One of them was a nutritionist, yoga master, meditation teacher and energy worker. There are two things that I still remember from the very first session with her. She said: "all is perfect", and "sit with the pain"

When I met Caroline Dupont, it was already December, 2007. She did an energy session on me that helped me a great deal with the back pain I was dealing with. Then we had a chat and at a given moment, after I had told her a little about my worries she said: "All is perfect. What is so horrible about that?" Even though I didn't understand fully it made me pause and think. Today I fully understand. It took me a while to accept things as they are; that they have their place in the whole and I should be conscious and responsible for my choices.

She also taught me to "sit with the pain" during meditation. This meant to sit quietly and feel the pain I was experiencing at a given moment with no agendas. Just be there with it.

The idea is that all energy looks for resolution so this pain or energy blockage that I was experiencing would go away in its own time.

I bought her CD "Open Heart Meditation" and started doing the practice, and I've got to tell you that it made a huge difference to me. My lower back pain was melting away! In January I took a whole day seminar with her and got some great tools to work with on blocked emotions, which I started using right away. She opened the doors to what I was suspecting was about to take place–if I allowed it–a transformation, a deep emotional healing. And I am very grateful for that.

Chi Gung Brings Revelation

The second person I met in another workshop was a nutritionist and a chi gung teacher, Angela Borgeest.

Every week she had a chi gung class for women. I attended for a while and then I continued doing this at home. When I first got started I didn't have a clue what to expect. I just wanted to have the experience to help my body heal. Little did I know that this was going to turn the key and push me over the edge to finally see clearly what was going on behind the scenes.

All this time I was doing lots of mental work (visualizations and affirmations), doing some deep breathing work, eating very healthy and more vegetarian and raw foods. Despite all this, I was still struggling with my digestive issues and losing weight.

In my very first class of chi gung (which is a martial art used for healing that involves deep breathing, deliberate movement and visualization) something that some would call "spooky" happened.

I had my eyes closed, following Angela's instructions and suddenly saw a vision of my mom, smiling at me. She looked so peaceful and loving. My mom had passed away in 1986.

As soon as I "saw" her, tears started to flow and I knew then that I still had lots of pain inside and perhaps other mixed emotions as well.

We discussed my experience with Angela and the rest of the group. She agreed that indeed there were things buried inside that needed resolution. Angela explained how, in Chinese medicine, each organ is associated with an emotion:

- Lungs are related to grief
- Heart to unconditional love
- Kidneys to fear
- Spleen and pancreas to courage
- Liver to anger

I kept on with my practice, which involved releasing emotions from those organs and incredibly enough each of them hurt at one time or another. Sometimes they all were hurting! It was very common for me to cry during the exercises by the way.

I was content anyway to know that I was allowing myself to let go of old emotions and unresolved issues. Things were coming out not only during the exercises but at any time. I was getting more and more insights that were helpful and revealing.

I kept absorbing information like a sponge, reading about energy medicine, nutrition and spirituality. Thanks to the fact that my business is related to natural health, the process of taking in all this info was easy and one thing was leading me to the next, and to the next, and to the next one. Then I started to find some clues and one of them was about…

Gluten Intolerance

When I read all about gluten intolerance and realized that I had the typical symptoms: heart burn, weight loss, malnourishment, muscle cramps, muscle pain, irritability, etc. I stopped having foods with gluten and oh boy! This made a huge difference to me.

My digestion improved, the cramps were less frequent and I started to feel much more energy. The pains and aches in my muscles and joints started to go away. Yuhuuu!! I felt on top of the world. I had found the answer, or so I thought.

Well, yes, life was looking good again but not for long. The dietary changes were helping but I was feeling gloomy, in limbo; feeling that I didn't fit anywhere; experiencing a feeling of loneliness that is beyond description. It's hard to put it into words. And it wasn't that I didn't have people who loved me a bunch. I did!

Until one day when…

I Got Instructions From The Divine

It was a cold morning at the end of January, 2008. Winter at its best! I was feeling quite restless, but did not know why. I was working at home, on the Internet, and suddenly it got disconnected. Odd thing, I thought. I tried to reconnect the Internet and nothing. I re-started the computer and nothing. Zippo. I really wanted to finish what I was doing and then go out to get some fresh air. I guess it had to do with this OLD idea of work first, play later, pfff. So, I tried one more time and nothing!! Grrrr! So frustrating!

So, I said to myself: OK. I'll go out now and will finish this later.

I got into the car not knowing where to go. I didn't have a plan, just wanted to be out! Took one of the main avenues near my home and immediately heard in my mind, loud and clear: Go to Akasha's Den.

What? I thought. It took me by my surprise but I'm a person who trusts my intuition and believes in angels and all that. So, I drove in the direction of this place and half way there I had a brilliant idea: I'll stop by the grocery store first. "NO!" said the voice in my head. And continued, "Go to Akasha's Den. NOW!"

Okay, okay… I did follow my inner voice, the voice of my guardian angel (or who knows) and went to this place where I had never been before. I knew where it was, that was all. I arrived, entered, browsed around and noticed that in the back of the store there were 5 women sitting in a small reading area, chatting, having tea, laughing, having fun. It felt great!

I moved up close listening to what they were saying and one of them invited me to sit down and join them. I did. I felt something very special going on. It felt like I had arrived at an important place. Their conversation was music to my ears. It was about emotional healing, health readings, mind power, spiritual growth, and all those topics that always, since I was little, have been so appealing to me.

At the very end of this spontaneous joining of the mini-gathering, one of the women approached me and asked me why I was there. That was enough to open the flood of tears that I had repressed and were ready to stream out. Tears started to roll down my cheeks and I barely managed to say, "I feel like I am drying up" … Wow, it makes me emotional even now as I remember it.

She took my hands, Deborah Filler is her name, and said: "I can help you". And then added, "Life doesn't have to be about suffering and struggling, you know?"

She handed me a business card and said, "Call me." Later that week I went to see her, got my first health and spiritual reading and then started a series of healing sessions with her that included hypnosis, Reiki, Erikson therapy and spiritual counseling. Deborah helped me immensely. She helped me to see how I could add more joy to my life at that moment, and encouraged me to continue exploring my life journey and all those lingering old issues. I was living what some would call the "darkest night of the soul" and I didn't have a clue!

With Deborah I cried and cried and started to feel like a human being again. She showed me that there was hope and that I was worthy of all I could dream in my life. Out of the blue she would call me to encourage me with loving and kind words. She was pivotal to me during this phase of my life and her love, patience, warmth and kindness are still fresh in my heart.

We worked on key family issues, especially the proper grieving of my mom, which somehow I hadn't allowed to happen when she passed away. I was a teenager and I guess I had thought I had to put on a straight face and act tough.

Medicinal Chi Gung & Master

During those months when I was seeing Deborah I knew of another excellent chi gung master who practiced a very specific type of energy healing through deep tissue massage. Her name was Master Teresa.

I discovered that a very experienced chi gung master would be able to transfer energy to you, and speed up the healing process, so I went to see her. That was precisely what I needed I thought. My energy levels were hitting their lowest point!

I saw her for almost three months. Again, it was a long drive to get to her office–about one hour–and at the end of every session I was flat exhausted. I couldn't wait to get home and lie on bed for a couple of hours at least.

My experience with Master Teresa was quite something. There was LOTS of pain involved. She could see where in my body the energy blockages were and worked on certain points that had "calcified". These points hurt like crazy every time she massaged them.

After the first session, which went for an hour, I remember driving home very weak. I was cold. My energy had plummeted and I was exhausted. When I got home I opened the door, went upstairs, crawled into my bed and slept for two hours or so. Next day things were different. I could feel the surge in my energy and thought, "It is working!" And it was. Thanks to her, I regained some precious energy.

She rescued me from the downward energy spiral I was embarking on. I couldn't understand what was happening. I was eating healthier foods than ever, taking enzymes, drinking green juices and still, there was something mysteriously wrong.

One of the things that Master Teresa said to me and I still remember is: "Things can wait. People can wait. Everything can wait. You are first!"

She didn't know me at all but could feel how big the word responsibility was for me. I think I'd been carrying this word on my shoulders with an inhuman heaviness since I was in 5th grade.

Until not long ago, I'd been working almost non-stop. The last four years had been about work, seminars, courses, tele-classes, you name it. Days of 14 to 16 hours at the computer were normal for me. Many months passed by like that and there were weeks in which I wouldn't put my feet on the street to take some fresh air because "I had so much to learn, to do, to implement, to accomplish." I wanted to succeed and help many people. Well, look where that got me!

I didn't understand that the first one that should be helped and cared for is oneself! My body had to say NO MORE, and make me stop. This was a big sign to me. I had to re-valuate things, let go of painful memories and old baggage that didn't serve me anymore, get connected again with my true self, take the time to love myself and allow myself to RECEIVE! Then I could restart with a new, fresh perspective.

As I mentioned before, I saw Master Teresa for almost three months and then I decided to look for someone closer to me. This brought me to my next step.

Acupuncture

My Korean friend, yes the same one, told me about a Korean doctor whom she was seeing. Soon I was seeing him too. I still had big digestion problems and my energy wouldn't stabilize. I had always believed so much in Chinese medicine so I bought 10 sessions with Doctor Sokjoo Sohn and started the treatments.

He said that my "Fire" or male energy was super low and that I had to do a deep cleanse. He gave me a mix of herbs he prepared specially for me and prescribed ginseng tea, which was like getting connected to a battery again. In less than a week I was riding my bicycle again, enjoying myself and my digestion was much better. I was feeling hungry again which was rare and sometimes eating bigger portions. I finished the ten sessions and continued my path that took me to a ...

Nutritionist

I was concerned with my weight. I knew there was something missing and up until now nobody had been able to find it. I already knew lots about nutrition but I knew I needed an expert to see if I could get to the bottom of this.

Another friend told me about Heather Grace whom she greatly recommended.

Heather is a nutritionist, energy worker, life coach and intuitive healer. She can feel and see things that many of us cannot, and according to my friend she was fabulous at clearing up things from this and past lives. It sounded interesting. Maybe I had something stuck in me from the time when I was a friend of Cleopatra... who knows!? I believe in past lives, old energies, etc. I was puzzled with what was happening to me and I was willing to take it to the end even if there were things that I couldn't understand with my human mind. I refused to believe that there was no answer. I always felt so confident that all was going to be all right.

Heather had psychic powers and did what we could call energetic healing combined with angel therapy. When I met Heather I thought that I already had had interesting experiences. Little did I suspect what was coming next!

In my very first session with Heather she surprised me with how much precision she talked about my pains and aches, my health situation and all that. Among the first things she said was that a…

Foreign Energy Was Attached to Me?

She called this "An energy" that didn't belong to me. She explained that sometimes there are energies wandering around lost and attach themselves to weak people to make a perfect host.

Anyhow, she described with all the details what and how I was feeling and said that this "foreign" energy was feeding off me and causing many of my health issues. Then she proceeded to perform a clearing of "this" energy with the help of the angelic realm which went on for three hours.

By the way, I'd been experiencing a very sharp pain above my heart toward the left side for months, something that nobody could diagnose and this pain intensified during the session. Lots of tears rolled down (just for a change) but after the session had finished, the pain was gone and best of all, it was gone forever! Heather said that the energy had been attached at that point and that with the help of the angelic realm, it had detached.

I went home feeling liberated, literally. The pain was gone and I had good appetite again, which by the way had become weak once more.

To this point, everything had worked but nothing had lasted, so my searching continued for the remaining pieces of the puzzle.

Liver Cleanse & Iodine for the Thyroid

The next step with Heather was to do a liver cleanse, a gentle one. I could feel the liver was a bit congested because it was painful. The cleanse consisted of eating veggies in any shape or form so I made lots of soups and steamed veggies and ate a bowlful every three hours or so for five days.

After the cleanse, my liver felt lighter. By that time I was eating lots of vegetables, raw foods, gluten-free foods, nuts and seeds, some cheese such as feta and cottage, as well as fresh and dried fruits. In general lots of vegetarian foods plus I was using my dehydrator to the max and loving it! I was still eating some eggs and seafood once in a while. It seemed that my digestion was getting better but progress was very slow—one step forward and two backwards. Still no weight gain.

Then I noticed that my hair was falling out in handfuls, I was colder than ever and still losing weight. I suspected I had something going on with my thyroid, perhaps an episode of low thyroid function. I had pretty much all the symptoms except the weight gain. A blood test said it was OK. I decided to do the home temperature test and it showed that it was a bit below the normal range.

Heather told me to do the home test for iodine deficiency and I turned out to be iodine deficient so I started taking iodine in drops. My energy levels went up and the hair loss diminished drastically. At the same time I also was taking a very good whey mineral matrix which I think was helpful as well. I learned about this product through the books of one of my favorite nutritionists, Dr. Bernard Jensen whose nutritional principles I was applying.

Heavy Metal Detox

Five weeks passed and I went to see Heather again. But the day before, I had an interesting experience. Something made me go to the health food section of the supermarket and my hand happened to be drawn to a product called "Spirulina". It suddenly hit me that perhaps the symptoms I was having could be the result of toxins and going through a heavy metal cleanse would help everything else I was already doing. When I got to Heather's, the first thing she mentioned was that she thought it important for me to have a heavy metal cleanse!!! So, of course, this was going to be my next step." I hope this is the last one", I thought. So, for two and a half months I took lots of spirulina, whey mineral matrix, alfalfa/ginger supplements, Swedish bitters, enzymes, probiotics, omega 3s, and of course my iron supplement which was alcohol based. My iron levels were still low and had been low for a couple of years.

I finally started to gain some weight but still there was something not right. I could feel it. My energy was like a roller coaster, up and down, and my sleep was irregular again as well.

I went to see Heather once more after I finished this cleansing cycle with the feeling that this was going to be the last appointment with her. And it was. Her job was done and now I was on my own, she said. I continued my spiritual and mental practices and added more enzymes to help with digestion. Then, I got to meet a…

Intuitive Healer and Reflexologist

My friend Gail had been seeing a reflexologist for a year, Suzanne Jambor, who worked nearby. I don't know why I hadn't felt compelled to see her before but after some weeks of seeing Heather for the last time, I felt it was time to see Suzanne.

I started the treatment with her at the end of January 2009–one session a week for three weeks and thereafter one session every two weeks. The first three weeks were very challenging. I would feel very rested and relaxed during the session but after a few hours it would be as if a train had run over me.

I wouldn't eat anything until next day because my body had no energy to digest anything, not even one leaf of lettuce. That meant about 20 hours without food. I thought that I was going to pass out (judging from my previous experiences with hypoglycemia) but I didn't. Again, another example of the body knowing better what it needs and is capable of adjusting to the circumstances.

Suzanne helped me immensely. I received her treatments throughout all of 2009 – and still see her sporadically. Her tiny office, out of a natural health food store, was a place of refuge to me. A small paradise filled with very calming, soothing, loving and healing energy.

She is one of the most caring, loving and giving persons I've ever met. She gave me great insights on the remaining emotional issues that were still blocking my healing process. I was fascinated by it all and continued to allow myself to clear, clear and clear. The journey had been very interesting indeed, and up to that moment there certainly had not been a single dull moment!

Of course, to not break the norm, I cried my eyes out with Suzanne.

On many occasions she took me back in time to very specific moments that helped me to pin point painful childhood memories and unresolved emotional issues that I still had to let go IF, and only IF I wanted to regain my strength, health and inner power.

The picture of my mom kept showing up as well as some memories of the time when I was around 9 and 11. Many of the things that I'd been pondering for a while were confirmed by Suzanne's strong intuition. I had the privilege of being raised by great parents who loved me deeply, protected me and always provided for me but as in any childhood there were things that seen through the eyes of a little girl were painful and distorted.

Suzanne suggested that I take Epson salt baths frequently to assist the clearing of emotional toxins. They helped indeed. I would feel very tired after our talks so I would take them before going to sleep – so lovely!

She also suggested for me to get rid of certain things that according to her carried a heavy, non-serving energy for me and which were "chaining" me to the old. They mostly were things I had brought from Colombia, where I was born. I was up for almost anything at this point in my life for the sake of my health and sanity so I followed her suggestion.

I don't know if this was symbolic, like a ritual I had to go through to help me even further or, if these things were really negatively charged for me. In any event I did it and felt good about it.

Maybe it had to do more with letting go; maybe it was about testing my commitment and making the statement that more than ever I was ready to do whatever was necessary. One of the things I'd been practising (and still do) is detachment, and what better opportunity to show it to the universe!

Choose: Live or Die

They say… what doesn't grow dies.

I remember one time, when I was at home alone, sitting on the couch in the living room, sooo tired, feeling disconnected from the world (and myself), wearing my 88 pounds, simply breathing and contemplating the surroundings when a thought struck me like lightening:

"This is it! I can do this. I choose to live. We can get better, Monica. We can do it."

I was talking to myself which I had stopped doing for a while. I knew that I was about to turn the corner. I felt like dying inside and knew that if I went below those 88 pounds things were going to get really tough. I had to make a decision so I did it.

This happened a couple of weeks after I finally got the answer to this health mystery. I think that I didn't want to accept what I had come to know because it meant so many things such as: another cleansing, another diet, letting go of other foods including fruits which I luuuved, and I suppose that subconsciously I knew that I'd have to let go much, much more than just certain foods.

There were still some destructive behaviors lingering around, clinging to my little human self but, I had to step up with my big human part and do something, otherwise the game was going to continue and most likely become uglier. Part of the answer was…

Candida Overgrowth

Yep. It's called candida albicans. By March, 2009, I was suspecting that what was causing my physical symptoms was a case of candida overgrowth.

It didn't surprise me in one way because in the past I had had many yeast infections. And something was getting worse and worse at this point, which is a strong signal of candida overgrowth: huge cravings for sweets, nuts, dry fruits and the like. I remember one night I didn't stop eating dry dates until I had finished a box of twelve! THAT had become an unusual behavior for me and had not manifested itself since I was in my 20's. But on the other hand why had I not connected this before? At first, I didn't understand this symptom and later I just "ignored" it, perhaps subconsciously because I didn't want to listen, I didn't want to assume responsibility, as simple as that.

Well, a couple of weeks went by and I saw Suzanne again. Her sessions were very helpful, but I still had lots of ups and downs and she was puzzled by it. While working on my feet she said, "You know what? It is as if you are…

"Sabotaging Yourself!..There is something strange going on here", she added.

"Oh, oh", I thought. That was exactly what I was thinking. I was also asking myself, "Why do I want to sabotage myself now that I think I know what this is all about?"

I had thought of candida. Yep. I had all the typical symptoms and a long history of antibiotic intake behind me. When I was a kid until my early twenties I had all sorts of infections: ear infections, sinus infections, colds, yeast infections.

While I was thinking about all this Suzanne added, "Could it be sugar related?" "Ha!" I exclaimed (I couldn't keep quiet anymore.) So then I told her that that was exactly what I had been thinking because of the symptoms I was experiencing. That same day, after the treatment, I got a supplement called "CandiGone" and felt very motivated to start the treatment to eradicate candida and claim my health back once for all! After dinner and before going to bed I took my first dose of what was going to change my life. Little did I know that doing it just like that (when the candida is chronic) can feel almost lethal!

That night I had the worst night I have ever had in my entire life. Seriously, I felt that I was in an inferno; maybe I had fever. My joints were aching; I could feel them throbbing non-stop. My whole back was in pain, every muscle, every tissue, every vertebra. I tossed and tossed, changed positions, prayed, visualized healing light and meditated all night. I talked to myself like never before and hoped to see the dawn soon. That night was eternal to me. I thought, "What have I done?"

Next day I got up feeling a deep pain all over my body. I knew that it had been too much for me, that I should have started slowly. Why hadn't they told me this at the store? Nothing like firsthand experience, eh?

My First Candida Diet

I did this treatment for a month and at the same time stopped eating many things such as sweets, fruits, starches and most dairy products. I was still eating a bit of feta and cottage cheese, plain yogurt, Ezekiel tortillas once in a while, and legumes once or twice a week.

Amazingly enough, after the first week, I started to sleep through the night. I was waking up with no muscle pain and my lower back pain was receding too. BINGO!!! I got it, I thought. And yes, I have figured it out. Things were getting better for me. I was getting results fast and felt that I was on the right track – finally! A month passed by and I was happy with the overall situation but intuitively I knew that I had to be more strict with the diet IF I really wanted to achieve full results – in less time. I had the idea that some of the foods I was eating were not that great so I continued my research until I found a strict candida diet which became the one I followed for more than a year. It was put together by Bee Wilder who had Candida for many years.

I cut out all dairy (except butter), starchy veggies such as carrots and beets, and legumes. I slowly cut down the quarter cup of rice I was having and the buckwheat flour I was using. Little by little, I started to add coconut oil until I got to 6 TBS a day, spread out, and added foods such as bone broth and sauerkraut (home-made), to help with digestion and assimilation. I started to eat more eggs and other good protein and that is when I invented a recipe for zucchini and spaghetti squash bread/muffins to satisfy my cravings for something sweet with a bread texture. (To make this exotic bread I used to shred the zucchini with a mandolin or food processor, arrange the long spaghetti-like strips on a tray and put it in the dehydrator. After 15 hours or so they were very dry so I could crunch them and make very small flakes that I used as "flour". I would combine a cup of this with 3 or 4 eggs and a bit of baking powder and bake it in the oven in a an oiled bread Pyrex or muffin tins. Mhh.. delish!)

I also added some new supplements such as calcium, magnesium, vitamin A, C and E, B-vitamins, and niacin. I continued with cod liver oil and discontinued the alcohol-based iron supplements and the Swedish bitters because alcohol also feeds candida!

I realized that all the vegetarian and raw foods I was eating were aggravating the candida situation! (My breakfast since then, May 8, 2009, has been eggs and lots of vegetables, most of the time sautéed or steamed and sometimes in salads.) I had done it the hard way, as I learned later on because I made most of the changes very fast. Most people take between 3 to 5 months to implement all these changes and I did it all in just over two, which means that I got the symptoms of the candida to die off big, big time!!

Candida Die Off Symptoms! 78+ Toxins Leaving In A Hurry

Remember the joint, muscle and back pain and aches I had? Well, they magnified I don't know how many times. It was awful! The fatigue and exhaustion became extreme. The irritability and mood swings–worse than ever. A roller coaster out of control! My sleep was better at times but not as good at others. If before I was crying because an old childhood memory crossed my mind now I was crying because a bug was passing by! I was hyperventilating more often and for longer periods of time. I was feeling more anxious than before and way more restless. Fortunately I knew that all was very normal and part of the candida cleanse. I just had to put up with it. The thing is that when candida dies it releases more than 78 toxins and the body feels it.

This part of the process lasted for about three months and then I started to feel a turnaround. As you can imagine I didn't have the energy or motivation to do many things during those three months and I was really blessed to have enough time to look after myself. This was the time to do that, to embrace it and accept it.

Cravings Assault

During those first three months I was hit by huge cravings quite often. In the beginning I thought that it was solely part of the candida die-off process because it is normal that candida, trying to hang on to what feeds it (sugary and high in carbohydrates foods) makes you feel that "you have to have those foods" otherwise you are going to perish. But as time passed and I started to get insights and aha moments, I started to realize that candida was acting more like an interim façade, hiding deeper unresolved issues within me. And then the real fun started!–the emotional rollercoaster and the deep healing my body, mind and soul had been waiting for.

All Happens For A Reason

I feel more than ever that there are no coincidences in life. I'm grateful for what these experiences have brought to my life. I would never have become who I am and continue to become without them.

These circumstances helped me to face many of my fears, old hurts and past conditionings and to re-discover my true self, claim my self-worth and zest for life. It taught me to love myself with compassion, to accept my dark and luminous sides, to let go all of that which was unserving and blocking my evolution. It also taught me to be patient with myself and not to take myself so seriously! I believe that it made me stronger, a more balanced and integrated person.

In The End The Answer Lies In Choosing Life!

This journey filled with ups and downs (and sometimes very, very flat times), has brought me here today, with you, back to my normal weight, wearing size 6 and having fun once more.

I learned and experimented with all sorts of techniques and practices, among them:

- meditation
- chi gung
- visualization
- reflexology
- breathing exercises
- angel therapy
- energy therapy
- hypnosys
- reiki
- ho'oponopono
- accupuncture
- nutritional therapy
- supplementation

In the end, I understand that the real key to true healing lies in loving yourself unconditionally, in trusting yourself and letting go. In choosing life above all and in everything and anything that honors your true self and allows your soul to shine through! So the question I have for you, now that we have crossed paths and you seem to be looking for some answers is...

Are You Ready to Change?

Are you ready to unload the past and let go all its wrinkled ghosts? Are you ready to open up your heart, allow self-love to expand in you and heal yourself? Are you ready to embrace all what you are... the so called "good" and "bad"? Are you ready to establish a relationship with yourself that is loving, caring and balanced? Are you ready to enjoy ALL what life has to offer (even the cakes, ice creams and truffles) with no guilt, remorse or attachment? If you are ready, if you want to finally tap into your core being where instead of fear, trust resides, and in place of doubt unconditional love flows, please come with me because I am going to show you 20, fun ways to do precisely that. I have done it... you can too!